Wonderfoods

To Elspeth
from Rita,
after Arran, June 2007.

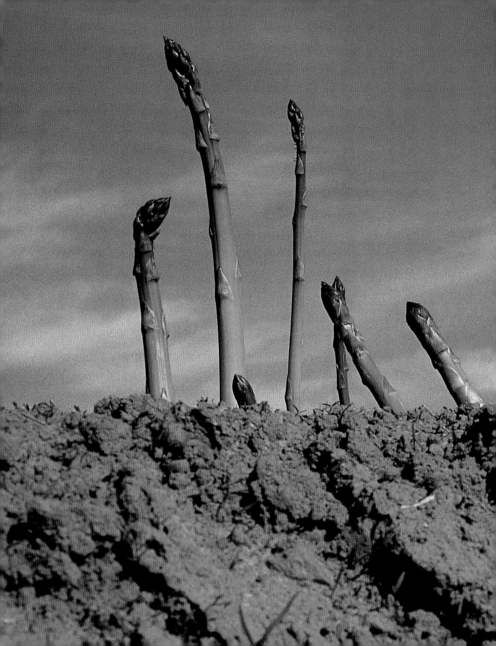

Wonderfoods

Natalie Savona

photographs by Jill Mead

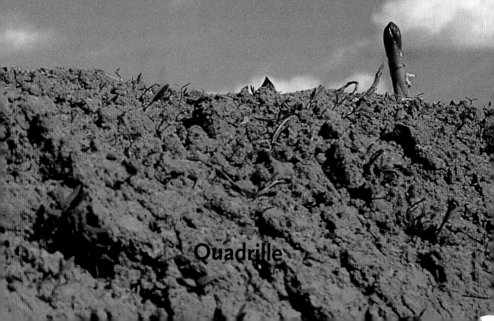

Quadrille

Dedication

This book is dedicated to those who have the privilege of choosing and producing wonderfoods, that they enjoy doing so and that they support those who do not have that choice.

This paperback edition
first published in 2006 by
Quadrille Publishing Limited
Alhambra House
27-31 Charing Cross Road
London WC2H 0LS

Reprinted in 2007
10 9 8 7 6 5 4 3 2

Text © 2006 **Natalie Savona**
Photography © 2006 **Jill Mead**
Design and layout © 2006 **Quadrille Publishing Limited**

Editorial director **Anne Furniss**
Creative director **Helen Lewis**
Project editor **Janet Illsley**
Senior designer **Ros Holder**
Photographer **Jill Mead**
Production **Ruth Deary**

Cataloguing in Publication Data: a catalogue record for this book is available from the British Library.

ISBN-13: 978 184400 441 6

Printed and bound in Singapore

Notes

Each wonderfood chapter is colour coded, as you will see from the contents list opposite. However many wonderfoods benefit several systems or areas of the body. The colour bars alongside the text introducing each wonderfood highlight other relevant areas.

All recipes serve 4 unless otherwise stated.

My measurements are casual, rather than meticulously precise. Spoon measures for dry ingredients – flour, spices etc – are rounded. Liquid measures are obviously level.
1 tsp = 5ml spoon; 1 tbsp = 15ml spoon.
I use a 300ml capacity mug to measure rice, grains etc.

I recommend you use fresh herbs, sea salt and freshly ground black pepper unless otherwise suggested.

I use medium eggs – ideally organic, otherwise free-range. I also recommend that you buy organic poultry.

Timings are for fan-assisted ovens. If you are using a conventional oven, increase the temperature by 10–15°C ($^1/_2$ Gas mark). Use an oven thermometer to check the temperature.

introduction

It is possible to thrive solely on the wonderfoods described in this book. Well, you'd need one addition for your health – water – and perhaps others every now and then for your soul, like cheesecake or coffee! But by and large, wonderfoods are abundant, easy to get hold of, and remarkably delicious. Even if not all are to your taste, many will be and you may even surprise yourself by starting to like new ones.

Pretty much all foods in their natural state would qualify as wonderfoods. Whoever designed them all did a very good job in packing them with what we need for fit, well bodies that will last us healthily into old age. The trouble is that we get diverted somewhere along the way to foods that challenge our bodies – ones that have been 'refined' to make them more appealing, a process that invariably takes some of the goodness away. Refined foods generally have sugar, fat, salt and chemicals added to them to make them taste 'better' or preserve them for longer.

There's certainly no harm in having such foods occasionally – a good quality pizza, a few glasses of wine and some ice cream are surely a good way to share food. But when such foods make up the majority of our diet – say after a day of toast and jam, biscuits, ham sandwich and crisps, fizzy drink, an apple, a chocolate bar – we become hooked. Even the seemingly healthier options, like a tuna sandwich or rice crackers instead of crisps, are often smothered in mayonnaise and salt. After such salty, sweet, fatty foods, a mound of steamed, green vegetables, plain grilled meat and brown rice seems boring to our palates and to our minds.

If you're reading this book, you're either already cherishing the deliciousness and goodness of wonderfoods or you are prepared to be inspired by them. You'll find you could fill your shopping basket just with wonderfoods and still not have bought two-thirds of those available.

Not all wonderfoods are necessarily wonderful for you though. Each of us is individual in terms of our nutritional needs and health conditions, not to mention our tastes. While a tomato, for example, is a rich source of the powerful antioxidants vitamin C and lycopene, for someone with arthritis it may trigger joint pain. Raw foods are always touted as wonderfully healthy and energising. Yet for a weak digestive system, raw food and whole grains are hard work. Although fruits are indisputably wonderfoods, in large amounts they can upset blood sugar and energy levels, and cause bloating. Most of us know what suits us and what doesn't; if you're not sure, it's best to consult a health professional to help you work out your ideal diet.

Selecting the entries for this wonderfoods book was easy enough – virtually all fruit and vegetables, herbs, whole grains, nuts, seeds and quality proteins qualify. The difficulty was whittling them down to fit into a reasonably sized book! At this stage, it became somewhat random – "If we've got broccoli, kale and cabbage, then perhaps the less popular Brussels sprout will have to go!" Then came the categorisation. This, too, took on a somewhat random turn after I'd listed all the things that each food was good for. Many wonderfoods fit into many categories. The colour bars alongside the information on each wonderfood guide you to other relevant categories – the contents list on page 6 provides the colour key. Garlic, for example, is in the Heart section, but it is also a good Immune and Detox food.

What didn't get into the book were 'extras' that you might add to foods, ingredients from health food shops such as wheatgerm, spirulina or brewers' yeast. All wonderful in themselves, but not quite foods as such...

Choosing your wonderfoods

Simply choosing to base your diet on wonderfoods is, in itself, a positive step. A good but very general guide on choosing your foods is this: if a food requires a label to tell you what is in it, think again about buying it. Even supermarkets sell most wonderfoods. On many levels, however, I prefer to buy my food at smaller shops such as local farm shops, independent health food shops and farmers' markets whenever possible. Eating locally grown, seasonal food should be a priority, though of course it isn't always available. After all, I love brown rice and pineapples, which I would never eat if I only bought Devon-grown produce!

From the point of view of chemicals used in growing food, organic produce is always the best choice. Even just a couple of organic items in your weekly shop is useful in helping to minimise your chemical exposure. But two points here...there is a good argument for having locally grown, non-organic food over organic varieties flown half way across the world and possibly farmed by underpaid workers. Secondly, just because something is organic, it doesn't mean it's good for you – organic cake and coffee, with organic milk and sugar is still a big hit on the sugar and stimulant front.

Preparing your wonderfoods

The recipes I have created here make use of as many wonderfoods as I could cram into each one and, you'll find, they are largely very simple to prepare. Even the recipes with longer lists of ingredients usually require only one pan or dish and very little effort.

You can rustle up a wonderfully tasty meal with just a few fresh ingredients as long as you keep a good stock of cupboard and fridge essentials, such as paprika, cayenne pepper, Chinese five spice, olives, peppercorns in a mill, a jar of tahini, garlic, stock powder such as Marigold, tamari (a type of soy sauce), Tabasco, Thai curry paste, miso paste, balsamic vinegar, cans of beans and chickpeas, cans of tomatoes and plenty of brown rice, oats, other grains, nuts and seeds.

A word about fats & sugar

I generally suggest using light olive oil for cooking as it is a monounsaturated fat. This means that it is chemically less susceptible to the damage from heat that affects sunflower and other seed oils, turning them into harmful trans fats. When you are softening onions or stir-frying, I recommend a method called 'steam-frying' which is pretty much the same thing but you use less oil and add a little water to stop burning or sticking. Butter does give a particular flavour to some recipes, but because it is high in saturated fat, it is best used sparingly, just for flavour. Blending it with olive oil also helps prevent it from burning.

Some recipes call for sugar and again, used sparingly, sugar is a perfectly reasonable part of a varied, healthy diet. Honey, maple syrup and molasses offer not only a different flavour from sugar but also a different nutrient base, though they are still, essentially, sugars. For this reason they are not valid substitutes for anyone who is avoiding sugar, such as a diabetic. One sugar substitute that I use very occasionally is xylitol, which sounds very chemical-like, but is a natural product extracted from plants. It looks and tastes like sugar but does not raise blood sugar levels in the same way, is lower in calories and helps prevent tooth decay.

My 'thing' on food

I was recently asked what my 'thing' was about food, what philosophy I espouse. And I'm often asked, "Do you believe in *x*, *y* or *z*?" regarding specific ways of eating such as veganism, raw food diet, high protein diet or whatever.

My 'thing' is to ensure that you eat a broad range of good quality foods and to enjoy what you eat. Do this, while being sensitive to what really works for you as an individual and that doesn't just mean for instant gratification. Just because your body is crying out for doughnuts every day at 11am, it doesn't mean they must be right for you. That said, I've seen far too many health-obsessed people control their diet to such a degree that the rigidity makes them irritable and ill and the odd doughnut would probably do them good. After all, there's no point worrying so much whether a food contains a little sugar if the worrying itself is going to give you an ulcer!

Food – preparing and sharing it – is, for those of us privileged to have the choice, one of life's joys and if you base what you eat on wonderfoods, you can't really go wrong.

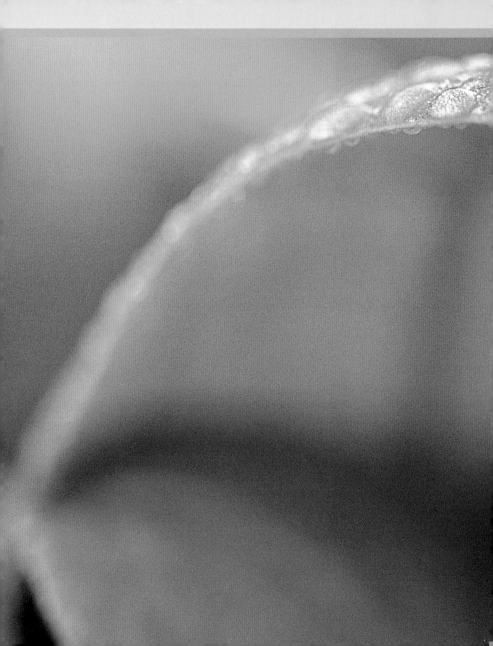

energy

The wonderfoods in this section are, indeed, packed with nutrients, starch and sweetness, which translate as energy that you can harness. They are of a variety that will leave you satisfied and, at the same time, provide you with good doses of important micronutrients – vitamins, minerals and other substances that are needed for countless uses in the body. The sure fire way of getting an instant hit of energy is to have a strong, sugary coffee or packet of sweets. That is, if you also want a sure way of crashing soon afterwards – setting up a vicious cycle of energy boost and exhaustion.

The body digests the sugars and starches within energy foods into sugar molecules that can be released into the bloodstream. The sugar is then carried around the body to cells where it is used to make energy. Quick-fix energy-giving foods, such as sweets or those made with refined (white) flour, are rapidly digested and released soon after eating into the bloodstream as sugar. Although this may seem like a good idea in the short-term, what goes up must come down. The body quickly responds to reduce rising blood sugar levels so you then feel a crash in energy, as well as in mood and concentration. The one thing that goes back up is your appetite... for another quick fix.

By contrast, energising wonderfoods contain fibre, fat, vitamins and minerals, which help regulate the rate at which they are converted into energy. So you still get a lift, but in a much more even, sustained way. You also get the vitamins and minerals that are involved in the actual conversion process to energy and other tasks around the body.

If you are consistently low in energy, you need to look at the whole of your diet, not just significantly boost your intake of the energy wonderfoods. You could try: making sure you have breakfast and evenly spaced meals throughout the day; not relying on quick fixes such as coffee, which are false friends; eating a variety of wonderfoods at each meal such as a banana with yoghurt and pumpkin seeds for breakfast, or sweet potato with chicken and broccoli for dinner.

You also need to ascertain and deal with the triggers for your tiredness. Insufficient sleep (obvious, but remarkably common), reliance on quick hits, low iron stores (common in vegetarians or vegans), over- or under-exercising, sluggish digestion and low moods can be causes of long-term fatigue. Whatever is going on for you, incorporating the wonderfoods in this chapter alongside others in the book, can go a long way to energising you.

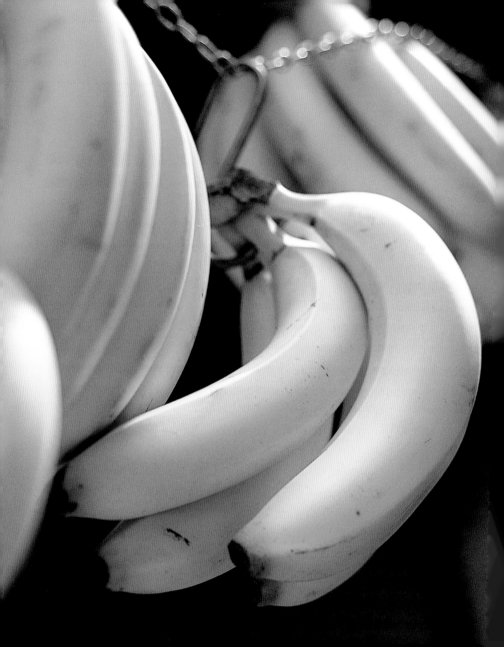

banana

Perhaps the ultimate fast food, bananas are understandably one of the most popular energy-boosters. A ripe banana is easy to digest as most of the starch has been converted to sugar, and can help relieve constipation (unripe ones may cause it). It is sugar combined with fibre that makes bananas so good for a sustained release of energy, even more so if eaten with some nuts or yoghurt. Fructo-oligo-saccharides (FOS) in bananas help feed 'good bacteria' in the gut. The pectin fibre in the fruit helps to soothe heartburn, ulcers or inflammation in the digestive tract, and to lower cholesterol. Bananas are also a good source of vitamin B6 and, like all fruits and vegetables, contain the mineral potassium. They also contain tryptophan, which the body can convert to serotonin – a hormone that helps lift moods and promote sleep. Multinational corporations cultivate vast swathes of former rainforest in Central and South America to produce cheap bananas, so buy Fair Trade bananas to support fairer, smaller producers.

almond baked bananas

A COMFORTING DESSERT THAT COMBINES COMPLEMENTARY TASTES AND TEXTURES.
USE BANANAS THAT ARE RIPE BUT FIRM.

4 **bananas**, peeled and
   sliced lengthways
8 **strawberries**, washed,
   hulled and halved
juice of 2 **oranges**
generous splash of amaretto
   liqueur
1 tsp butter
2 tbsp **almonds**, chopped
natural **yoghurt**, to serve

Preheat the oven to 180°C/Gas 4. Lay the bananas and strawberries in a baking dish. Pour the orange juice and amaretto over the fruit and dot with the butter. Sprinkle on the almonds and bake in the oven for 15–20 minutes until the bananas are soft.

Serve with a dollop of natural yoghurt.

frozen coco-nana

FROZEN BANANAS ALONE ARE LIKE AN ICE CREAM TREAT IN THEMSELVES — THIS
COMBINATION MAKES THEM EVEN BETTER.

4 **bananas**, peeled
1 tbsp shredded **coconut**
(ideally fresh, otherwise
use dried)
1 tbsp **sesame seeds**
100ml **coconut** milk
1 tbsp **honey**
juice of 1 **lime**
splash of rum (optional)

Chop the bananas into 2.5cm pieces, lay them
on a metal tray and put them in the freezer for
at least an hour.

In a dry frying pan, toast the shredded coconut
and sesame seeds until golden brown.

Just before serving, get the bananas out of the
freezer and whiz in a blender with the coconut
milk, honey and lime juice until smooth, adding
a splash of rum if you like.

Spoon into small serving bowls, top with the
toasted coconut and sesame seeds and serve.

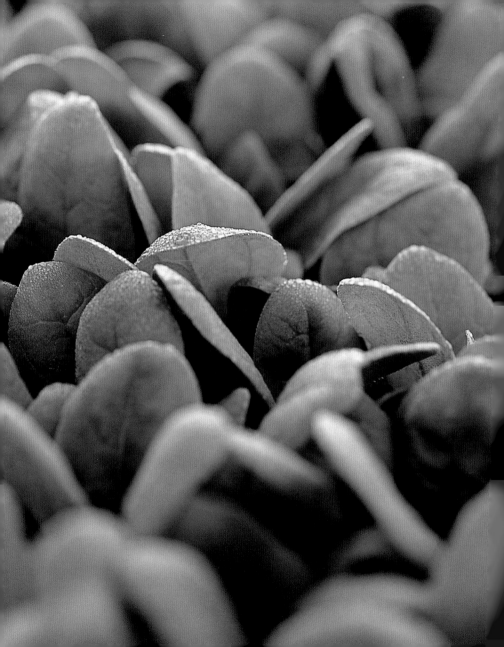

spinach

Spinach is perhaps best known for its iron content, thanks to Popeye, although the iron in spinach is not in its most accessible form to humans (compared with meat, for example). It is, however, a godsend for vegetarians and vegans, and a squeeze of lemon juice will provide vitamin C, which helps iron absorption. Iron is essential for healthy blood cells, enabling them to carry oxygen efficiently around the body for every cell to create energy – one of the first signs of being low in iron is fatigue. Spinach is also laden with other important nutrients such as calcium (150% more than milk, weight for weight), magnesium (a mineral 72% of British women are low in) and beta carotene, the vegetable form of vitamin A and a useful antioxidant. A substance called neoxanthin in spinach has been shown to help prostate health. Vitamin K, also contained in spinach, is important for bone health and blood clotting. The green in leaves, including spinach, comes from the chlorophyll, a substance that, along with the fibre, acts as a powerful 'cleanser'.

baby spinach tart

EVEN PEOPLE WHO AREN'T BIG FANS OF GREEN VEG USUALLY LOVE THIS CLASSIC
RECIPE. LEFTOVERS, IF THERE ARE ANY, ARE IDEAL FOR A PACKED LUNCH OR PICNIC.
SERVES 2

1 tbsp olive oil, plus extra
   to brush
2 medium **onions**, peeled
   and finely chopped
2 **garlic** cloves, peeled and
   crushed
300g **spinach**, washed and
   chopped
about 20 olives, stoned and
   chopped
1 tbsp finely chopped mint
1 tbsp finely chopped
   parsley
1 **egg**, beaten
200g feta cheese, finely
   crumbled
1 tbsp **sunflower seeds**
8 sheets of filo pastry

Preheat the oven to 180°C/Gas 4. Heat the olive
oil in a frying pan, add the onions and garlic and
cook over a low heat for about 5 minutes to soften.
Add the spinach and stir until it has wilted, then
tip the lot into a large bowl. Add the olives, herbs,
egg, feta and sunflower seeds, and toss to mix.

Layer the filo sheets in a 25cm flan dish,
leaving some overhanging the rim all round and
brushing each layer with olive oil. Pour the filling
into the filo case and roughly crumple the
overhanging pastry back up to edge the tart. Bake
in the oven for 30–35 minutes until the filling is set
and the filo is golden brown.

duck & spinach salad

THIS MAKES A SUPERB TASTY LUNCH OR SUMMER SUPPER — ONE TO IMPRESS
GUESTS. YOU COULD USE PAPAYA INSTEAD OF THE MANGO.

4 duck breast fillets, with
   skin
2 tsp Chinese five spice
   powder
sprinkling of cayenne
   pepper
250g baby **spinach** leaves,
   washed
1 **mango**, peeled and diced
handful of coriander leaves,
   roughly chopped
4 spring **onions**, trimmed
   and sliced
2 large, cooked **beetroot**,
   peeled and diced
1/3 long **cucumber**, chopped
juice of 1 **lime**
1 1/2 tbsp tamari or soy sauce
2 tbsp **sesame** oil

Preheat the oven to 180°C/Gas 4. Score the skin
side of each duck breast a few times and rub with
the Chinese five spice and cayenne pepper,
pushing some into the slashes to touch the meat.

Preheat a dry frying pan and quickly fry the
duck, skin-down, for about 5 minutes. Turn the
duck breasts and fry for a couple of minutes, then
place in an ovenproof dish and finish cooking in
the oven for about 10 minutes, depending on how
pink you like your meat and how thick the fillets
are. Rest in a warm place for 5 minutes.

Meanwhile, in a large bowl, toss the spinach
with all the other ingredients, then divide among
plates. Slice each duck breast and arrange on top.
Serve at once, while the duck is still warm.

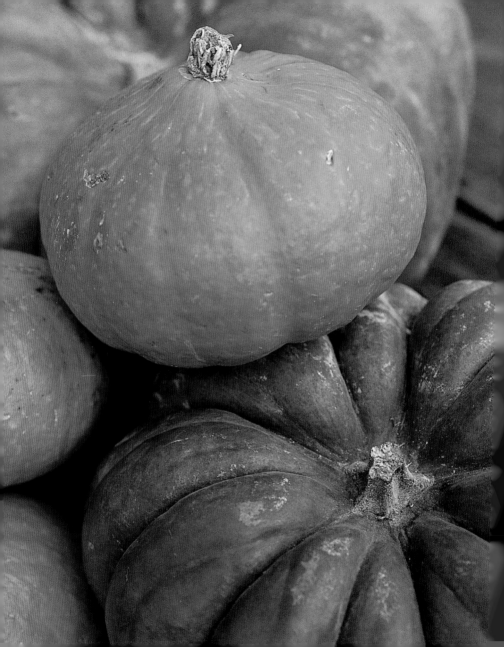

pumpkin &
squash

Native to the Americas, where it was originally used to make flour, the lowly pumpkin may be what got the first Pilgrims through their first winter in 1620. For those who count, pumpkin is remarkably low in calories, although its starch is good for energy. It was used as a folk remedy to kill intestinal worms, but not as effectively as its seeds. Pumpkin is high in fibre, which is useful for easing food through the intestines and helping clear waste. As its orange colour suggests, pumpkin contains beta carotene which, amongst other things, helps protect against the harmful rays of the sun. Halloween lanterns aside, the pumpkin and squash family comes in an array of shapes, sizes and colours, perhaps the most tasty being the butternut. They can be eaten roasted, mashed, in soups, stews, savoury and sweet pies or breads, even grated raw. Because pumpkin can be bland, many recipes add heaps of fat or sugar, but steer clear of those to get the gains from this versatile, filling vegetable.

butternut & feta salad

FRESH, RAW SPINACH OFFSETS COMFORTING WARM SQUASH AND CRUMBLY FETA
CHEESE PERFECTLY — FOR A SUBSTANTIAL LUNCH OR LIGHT DINNER.

1 small butternut **squash**,
    roughly cubed
1 **red pepper**, cored,
    deseeded and cut into
    squares
few **thyme** sprigs, or
    $^1/_2$ tsp dried
splash of olive oil
dash of balsamic vinegar
freshly ground black pepper
225g baby **spinach** leaves,
    washed
3 spring **onions**, trimmed
    and finely sliced
squeeze of **lemon** juice
8–12 cherry **tomatoes**,
    quartered
200g feta cheese, cubed

Preheat the oven to 180°C/Gas 4. Don't bother peeling the butternut for this but do scoop away the seeds. Put it into a roasting dish with the red pepper and thyme, plus generous dashes of olive oil and balsamic vinegar. Season with pepper, toss well and roast in the oven for about 40 minutes.

Meanwhile, pile the spinach equally on to four plates. Scatter the spring onions over, drizzle with a little olive oil and add a squeeze of lemon juice.

When the butternut and red pepper are cooked, leave to cool slightly, then mix in the tomatoes and feta. Pile the warm mixture on top of the spinach leaves and eat immediately. Delicious with warm, crusty brown rolls.

pumpkin & bacon soup

BACON MAY NOT BE THE HEALTHIEST OF FOODS, BUT ITS SALTINESS COMBINED WITH RATHER BLAND, SWEET PUMPKIN IS DELICIOUS. EATEN WITH WHOLEMEAL BREAD, THIS SOUP MAKES A SATISFYING MEAL IN ITSELF, OR YOU CAN SERVE IT AS A WARMING STARTER BEFORE A LIGHT MAIN COURSE.

*1 large wedge of **pumpkin**, or 1 large butternut **squash***
*1 large **onion**, peeled and finely diced*
*2 **celery** sticks, sliced*
a little olive oil
300–400g smoked bacon or gammon, diced
freshly ground black pepper
1 litre vegetable or chicken stock
*handful of **parsley**, chopped*

Peel and deseed the pumpkin or squash and cut into cubes. (The soup will be even sweeter and richer if you roast the pumpkin at this stage for 30 minutes at 180°C/Gas 4, but it's not essential.)

In a large, covered saucepan over a low heat, soften the onion with the celery in a little olive oil. Add the bacon and cook, stirring, for a few minutes until evenly coloured.

Add the pumpkin, season with pepper and then pour in the stock. Simmer, covered, until the pumpkin is soft, about 30 minutes depending on the variety (or much less if pre-roasted).

Whiz the soup briefly using a hand-held stick blender to purée some of the pumpkin and thicken the liquor, but keeping a chunky texture. Stir in the chopped parsley and serve as a thick, warming soup.

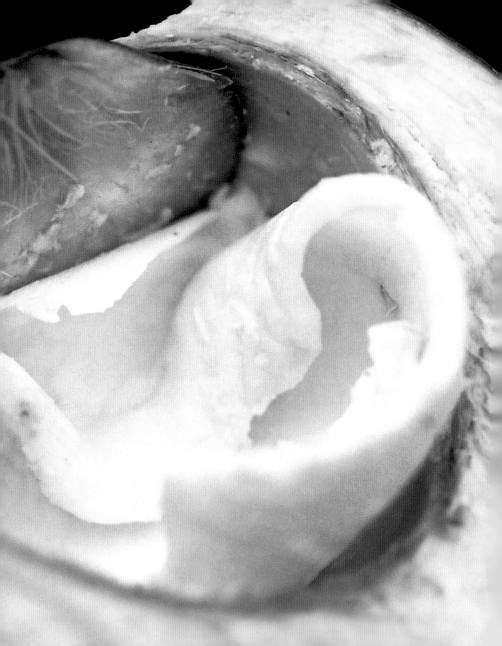

coconut

In India, coconut palms are considered a *kalpavriksha*, or tree of life and, indeed, pretty much every part of the plant is used. Although coconuts are one of the rare sources of saturated fat (SF) in plants, it's not all bad news. About half of a coconut's saturated fats are known as 'medium chain triglycerides' or MCTs, which seem to increase the burning of calories, i.e. they promote energy production and are not stored in the body as fat. So it seems coconut can actually help boost energy and weight loss. MCTs are also easily digested and absorbed, unlike other saturated fats. Coconuts are a rich source of an MCT called lauric acid (as is breast milk), which the body can convert into an antiviral and antibacterial substance called monolaurin. They also contain a little of the antifungal caprylic acid. Because it is high in SF, coconut oil is, like butter, good for cooking as it is not denatured by heat. But like all fatty foods, coconut should be eaten in moderation.

aromatic fish parcels

I FIRST TASTED THIS WHEN MY FRIEND, CHARMAINE, COOKED IT FOR DINNER ON A WINTER'S NIGHT IN A DORSET THATCHED FARMHOUSE. NOT VERY ENGLISH BUT WARMING ALL THE SAME, ESPECIALLY WHEN SERVED WITH BROWN RICE AND STEAMED VEGETABLES.

4 **fish** fillets, such as
   haddock or snapper
2 lemongrass stalks, sliced
2 **garlic** cloves, peeled and
   sliced
2–3cm piece fresh root
   ginger, peeled and sliced
1 chilli, deseeded and finely
   sliced (more if you like
   it hot)
2 **limes**, halved
1 small can **coconut** milk

Preheat the oven to 180°C/Gas 4. Cut four large pieces of greaseproof paper and fold each one in half – folded, they need to be big enough to enclose a fish fillet with enough paper to scrunch up over the top to seal.

Lay a fish fillet in the middle of each double piece of paper. Scatter the lemongrass, garlic, ginger and chilli over and under the fish fillets and squeeze the juice of $1/2$ lime over each one. Fold up the sides of the paper, then drizzle about 2 tbsp coconut milk on each fillet.

Bring the edges of the paper together over the fish, then roll and scrunch them together, tucking in the ends to form little parcels. Place on a baking tray and bake for about 15 minutes, depending on the thickness of the fillets.

Serve the fish in their parcels on warm plates, with stir-fried vegetables and brown rice.

mango with coconut rice

APRIL IN THAILAND, STALLS AT THE SIDE OF THE ROAD PILED HIGH WITH RIPE
MANGOES…IT'S ALL YOU CAN DO TO RESIST HAVING SERVING AFTER SERVING OF
THIS DELICIOUS, RICH DISH.

150g **brown rice** (or Thai
   fragrant)
3 tsp **sesame seeds**
200ml **coconut** milk
40g sugar or alternative
   equivalent (see page 10)
2 ripe **mangoes**, peeled and
   sliced off the stone

Cook the rice according to the packet directions,
depending on the type you use – ideally go for
brown, if not, Thai fragrant rice.

Meanwhile, in a dry frying pan over a medium
heat, toss the sesame seeds until they start to pop
and then set aside to cool.

When the rice is cooked, drain if necessary,
then add the coconut milk and sugar and stir over
the heat for about 10 minutes until you have a
thick, mass of rice that's sticky but not runny.

Allow the rice to cool a little before serving in
small bowls, topped with slices of fresh mango
and sprinkled with the toasted sesame seeds.

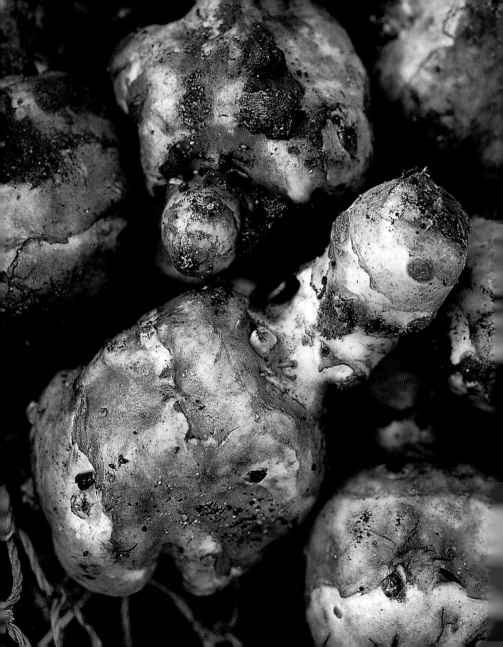

jerusalem
artichoke

Jerusalem artichokes are not remotely related to the more familiar globe artichokes and they have nothing to do with Jerusalem. In fact, they are a member of the sunflower family and are sometimes called sunchokes. The tubers have a delicate, nutty flavour and can be used similarly to potatoes: boiled, steamed, mashed, in soups, baked or fried, but also raw. Unlike potatoes, sunchokes provide a gentle release of their energy because they store it as inulin rather than sugar. So they are a good food for people with diabetes or poor blood sugar balance. It is the soluble fibre, inulin, that gives them their notoriety for inducing wind because it is a 'prebiotic' i.e. it feeds the good bacteria in the gut. A plus point is that inulin can bind with waste products or toxins, helping to escort them out of the body. Studies have shown that inulin can help to lower cholesterol levels, too. Jerusalem artichokes also contain good amounts of iron – weight for weight, even more than lean beef.

jerusalem chicken

THIS A BEAUTIFULLY FLAVOURED DISH FROM THE MIDDLE EAST. ALTHOUGH THE
NAME OF THE VEGETABLE SUGGESTS THAT IT ORIGINATES FROM THIS REGION, IT IS
NATIVE TO NORTH AMERICA AND RELATED TO THE SUNFLOWER. JERUSALEM
ARTICHOKE IS THOUGHT TO BE A CORRUPTION OF *GIRASOLE*, THE ITALIAN WORD
FOR SUNFLOWER, MEANING 'TURNING TO THE SUN'.

2 tbsp olive oil
*4 tbsp **lemon** juice*
*10 **garlic** cloves, peeled and halved*
*200g **Jerusalem artichokes**, peeled and sliced*
*10 **cardamom** pods*
*6 saffron threads (or ¹/₂ tsp ground **turmeric**)*
freshly ground black pepper
*8 **chicken** thighs (or drumsticks if you prefer)*
*12–15 **basil** leaves*
2 tbsp pine nuts, lightly toasted

In a large saucepan, mix the olive oil and lemon
juice, then add the garlic, Jerusalem artichokes,
cardamom, saffron and some pepper. Add enough
water to cover the artichokes and bring to the boil.
Add the chicken pieces, stir, then cover and
simmer gently for an hour.

Just before serving, stir in the basil leaves and
scatter over the pine nuts. Serve with brown rice
and a steamed green vegetable, such as spinach.

jerusalem artichoke bake

THIS IS A SLIGHTLY HEALTHIER VERSION OF THE TRADITIONAL DAUPHINOISE,
WHICH IS USUALLY MADE WITH POTATOES AND LASHINGS OF CREAM. IT GOES WELL
WITH ANY MEAT OR CHICKEN DISH.

300g **Jerusalem artichokes**, well scrubbed and thinly sliced
300g celeriac, peeled and thinly sliced
1 **onion**, peeled and finely sliced
1 **garlic** clove, peeled and crushed
200ml vegetable or chicken stock
200ml soured cream
freshly ground black pepper
pinch of freshly grated nutmeg
1 **egg**
handful of grated Gruyère cheese

Preheat the oven to 180°C/Gas 4. Layer the Jerusalem artichokes, celeriac and onion in a shallow ovenproof dish, sprinkling with the garlic.

Mix the stock with the soured cream, season with pepper and nutmeg and beat in the egg. Gently pour this mixture over the vegetables and top with the cheese. Bake for around 40 minutes, checking whether the vegetables are cooked through after about 30 minutes by poking a skewer into the middle.

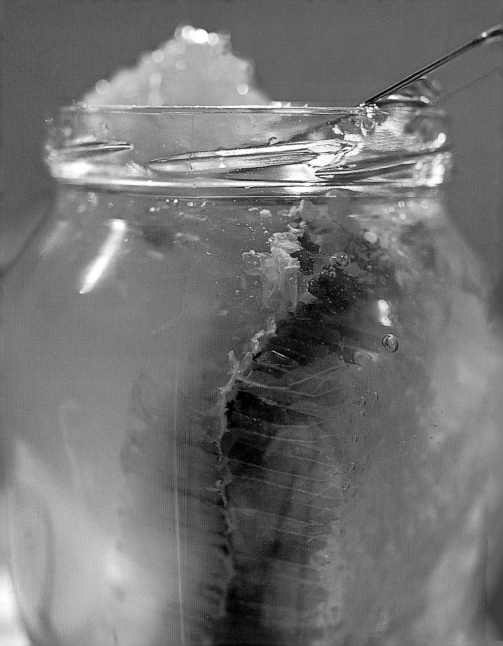

honey

Reputed to be the food of the gods, honey has even crept into our language to mean love. It is 97% sugar and primarily a source of energy that is easily absorbed by the body. For this reason, it shouldn't be used excessively or on its own, otherwise it contributes to tooth decay, weight gain and even diabetes. To get more than just a unique sweetener – and the best of that remaining 3% – it's essential to eat raw honey, harvested by scrupulous beekeepers who do not allow medication or sugar to contaminate their product. The qualities of the honey also depend on the flowers from which the nectar came – for example, manuka honey from New Zealand has the antiseptic properties of the manuka tree. Raw honey contains residues of propolis – a resin-like substance made by bees with healing and antimicrobial properties – used for centuries on the skin to treat burns, wounds and ulcers. Another natural sweetener containing valuable nutrients, especially iron and other minerals, is blackstrap molasses, a by-product of refining sugar.

honeyed granola

THIS RECIPE MAKES A BIG BATCH OF CEREAL THAT CAN BE STORED IN A SEALED CONTAINER FOR A MONTH OR SO.

500g rolled **oats**

2 tbsp **sunflower seeds**

2 tbsp **pumpkin seeds**

2 tbsp **almonds** or hazelnuts, roughly broken

2 tbsp dried shredded **coconut**

8 tbsp **honey**

8 tbsp **coconut** oil or olive oil

2 tsp vanilla extract

3 tbsp raisins, sultanas or dried berries

8 dried **apricots**, finely chopped

Preheat the oven to 160°C/Gas 3. Line a large shallow baking tin with greaseproof paper.

In a large bowl, combine the oats, seeds, nuts and coconut. In a small saucepan, heat the honey, oil and vanilla extract. Just before the mixture boils, pour it over the dry ingredients and mix well.

Spread the mixture out in the prepared tin and bake for about 25 minutes, stirring it halfway through cooking. As soon as you take it out of the oven, add the dried fruit and toss to mix.

Leave the granola to cool completely before storing it in an airtight container. Eat a bowlful for breakfast, with milk or soya milk.

honey grilled salmon

THIS HAS A LOVELY SMOKEY BARBECUE FLAVOUR. THE MARINADE ALSO WORKS
WELL ON CHICKEN OR LAMB.

4 fresh **salmon** *steaks or fillets*
FOR THE MARINADE
2 tbsp **honey**
1 tsp smoked paprika
1/2 tsp Tabasco sauce
1 tbsp cider vinegar
2 tsp tamari or soy sauce

Mix the marinade ingredients together in a large bowl. Add the fish steaks and swish them around so they are well coated. Leave to marinate for about 20 minutes.

Preheat the grill and grill the salmon steaks, basting frequently with the marinade, until cooked to your taste. This should take no longer than 3 minutes each side, depending on the thickness of the fish. If you are cooking fillets with skin, grill skin-side up for around 4 minutes, then turn and cook flesh-side up for about 1 minute only.

Serve with a steamed green vegetable, such as broccoli or kale.

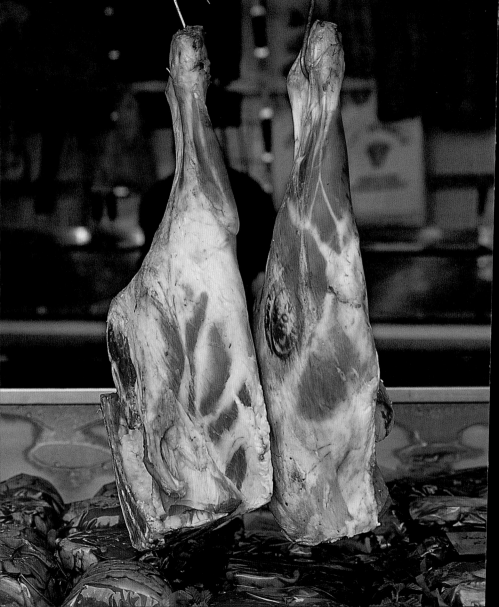

lamb

Red meat is often maligned for its saturated fat and cholesterol and yes, we should keep those to a minimum, but lean meat such as lamb (or even beef), can be a wonderful addition to a menu. The prime cuts from naturally reared, active animals that graze in fields are generally lean – so you get the goodness with minimal saturated fat and cholesterol. Red meat is an excellent source of protein and easily absorbed iron – more so than any vegetable source of this vital mineral. Iron is fundamental for carrying oxygen throughout the body efficiently, for cells to make energy. Many menstruating women end up low in iron, so eating red meat, such as lamb, is a useful way of avoiding this. Energy-wise, a protein-rich meal is more sustaining and lamb is also rich in B vitamins used for, amongst countless other things, making energy inside our cells. Unlike plant foods, red meat is a particularly good source of vitamin B12, which is needed for good moods and a healthy heart.

lamb curry kebabs

YOU COULD APPLY THIS MARINADE TO ANY MEAT, FISH OR PRAWNS, BUT LAMB TAKES ON ALL THE SPICES PARTICULARLY WELL. FOR OPTIMUM FLAVOUR AND FRAGRANCE, USE WHOLE CUMIN AND CORIANDER SEEDS, TOAST THEM IN A DRY FRYING PAN UNTIL THEY RELEASE THEIR AROMA, THEN GRIND TO A POWDER.

1kg lean, boned **lamb** (ideally leg), cubed
FOR THE MARINADE
1 medium **onion**, peeled and finely diced
3 **garlic** cloves, peeled and crushed
1 tbsp olive oil
3 tbsp **lemon** juice
freshly ground black pepper
2 tsp ground cumin
1 tsp ground coriander
1 tsp paprika
2 tbsp grated **coconut** (ideally fresh, otherwise use dried)
3 tbsp natural **yoghurt**
TO SERVE
handful of coriander leaves

Mix all the marinade ingredients together in a large bowl. Add the meat and stir well to coat all the pieces thoroughly. Leave to marinate for at least an hour, ideally 4 or 5 hours.

Preheat the grill or barbecue. Thread the meat on to four long skewers. Grill the meat skewers under a high heat, or cook on the barbecue, turning them occasionally, until browned on all sides but still pink in the middle. Allow 10–12 minutes, or longer if you prefer.

Scatter with coriander and serve with Scented savoury rice (page 67), Apricot salsa (page 175) and a Wonderfoods green salad (page 111).

grilled lamb with minty tomato salsa

MAKE A BIG BOWL OF THIS SALSA TO GO WITH BARBECUED MEAT IN LATE SUMMER,
ESPECIALLY IF YOU FIND YOU HAVE LOTS OF GREEN TOMATOES IN THE GARDEN.

4 **lamb** steaks or chops
FOR THE TOMATO SALSA
3 large, green **tomatoes**,
    roughly chopped
2 tbsp chopped mint
1 tbsp chopped **parsley**
1/2 small red **onion**, peeled
    and very finely chopped
1 small **garlic** clove, peeled
    and crushed
1 tbsp olive oil
juice of 1/2 **lemon**
freshly ground black pepper

Put all the ingredients for the tomato salsa in a serving bowl and toss to mix.

Preheat the grill or barbecue. Cook the lamb steaks for about 3–5 minutes each side until nicely browned on the outside but still pink in the middle, or until they are done to your taste.

Serve with the tomato salsa and Herby sweet oven chips (page 198).

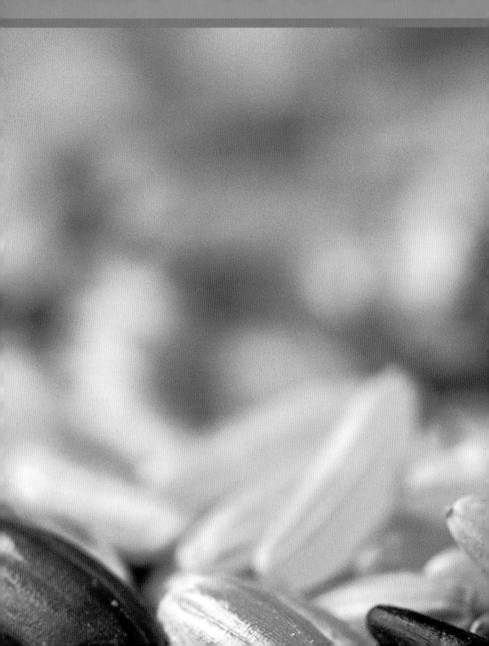

digest

Given that the digestive tract is a long tube comprising different parts, each with their different jobs, there's a long list of essentials for keeping it working efficiently and comfortably. Not to mention the differences between individuals, whether it's a case of not 'going' often enough, 'going' too regularly, a tendency to heartburn, or being able to eat anything...The wonderfoods here offer a range of qualities in soothing the gut. It's a matter of finding out what works for you as an individual.

One of the most common of all digestive complaints is constipation. This can be tricky to resolve, but the solution can be as simple as eating more vegetables and fruit, like apples. The fibre in these, as in whole grains (such as brown rice and buckwheat), seeds and pulses, helps bulk out the stool, making it easier to pass. That said, the inherent indigestibility of pulses and the high sugar content of fibre-rich dried fruit make some people bloated and congested – a prime example of our individuality. Another key ingredient for regularity is water, to prevent the stool from becoming dry and impacted in the colon and difficult to pass.

For digestive processes to work smoothly, food needs to be eaten slowly, in manageable quantities and at reasonable intervals. Chewing well and pausing between mouthfuls is the right start. This ensures that the food is mechanically broken down and stimulates the release of digestive juices in the stomach and intestines – gearing the whole system up to process the food well. The more efficiently this happens, the more nutrients you get out of your food and the less likely you are to have digestive difficulties like indigestion or wind. Some foods, such as papaya and pineapple, contain enzymes that actually help the breakdown of food into smaller particles. The spices in this section have been used as digestive aids for many, many years.

Another potential complication with the digestive system is negative reactions to particular foods. There is an increasing awareness that some people do not tolerate certain foods well. Specific foods give them indigestion, bloating, flatulence, constipation, diarrhoea, or even symptoms that are seemingly unconnected to the gut, such as lethargy or eczema. The wonderfoods in this section are generally fine for most people. Common culprits are wheat (or gluten, which is found not only in wheat but also in oats, rye and barley), dairy products and soya. This is a very individual matter that should be explored with a health professional so as not to restrict the diet dangerously or unnecessarily.

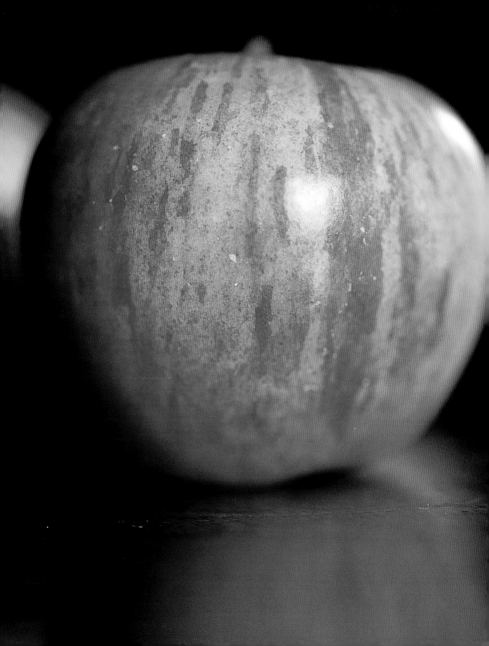

apple

Throughout history apples have symbolised love and fertility, though it's easy to cast them aside in favour of exotic fruits, especially given the bland taste of many common apples these days. But make careful choices and you could barely do better. Apples contain pectin, a soluble fibre that gently but efficiently cleanses the intestines, binding with waste products and escorting them out of the body. It also encourages the proliferation of beneficial bacteria in the gut, helps keep cholesterol down and helps balance blood sugar levels. Apples are a source of quercetin, which helps protect cholesterol from damage that causes a build up in arteries. They are easily digestible, alkaline and about 85% water – so hydrating too. Malic acid is found in apples and this plays a role in all human cells as part of the energy production process. Choosing tasty apples can be hit and miss, so you need to experiment – at farmers' markets and farm shops you are more likely to have unusual, flavourful varieties.

mackerel with apple purée

I FIRST MADE THIS WHEN WE HAD MASSES OF APPLE PURÉE IN THE FRIDGE AFTER PICKING APPLES AT A FRIEND'S ORCHARD IN DEVON. COMBINED WITH THE HORSERADISH, THE PURÉE MAKES A SHARP CONTRAST TO THE OILY FISH.

2 large cooking **apples**, quartered, cored and peeled
grated zest of 1 **lemon**
3 tbsp water
4 **mackerel**, gutted, heads on
2 heaped tsp horseradish sauce

Roughly chop the cooking apples and put them into a saucepan with the lemon zest and water. Cover and cook slowly until the apples are soft and pulpy.

Preheat the grill. Score the mackerel two or three times on each side and cook them under the hot grill for about 8 minutes, turning halfway through. Really fresh fish can be left slightly underdone.

Mix the horseradish into the warm apple purée. Serve the mackerel with a generous spoonful of spiked apple purée on the side.

apple custard tart

THE INSPIRATION FOR THIS TART IS A COUPLE OF DIFFERENT RECIPES FROM THE WONDERFUL MOOSEWOOD COOKBOOK BY MOLLIE KATZEN. THE BASE HAS A CRUNCHY COURSE TEXTURE. I SOMETIMES MAKE A FINER CRUST BY GRINDING THE OATS IN A BLENDER FOR A MINUTE OR SO BEFORE I START.

FOR THE BASE
100g rolled **oats**
50g hazelnuts, chopped
30g **sunflower seeds**
1 tbsp brown sugar or
    alternative equivalent
    (see page 10)
pinch of salt
1 tsp ground **cinnamon**
80g butter, melted
FOR THE FILLING

3 **eggs**
300g natural **yoghurt**
50g brown sugar or
    alternative equivalent
    (see page 10)
2 tsp vanilla extract
1 tsp ground **cinnamon**
2 large cooking **apples**

Preheat the oven to 180°C/Gas 4. For the base, mix the oats, nuts, seeds, sugar, salt and cinnamon together in a large baking tray and toast in the oven for about 30 minutes.

Meanwhile, prepare the filling. In a bowl, whisk together the eggs, yoghurt, sugar, vanilla extract and cinnamon. Peel, core and slice the apples.

Stir the melted butter into the oven-toasted base ingredients and press the mixture into a deep 20cm flan dish. Lay the sliced apples on the base and carefully pour the filling mixture over them. Bake for 35–40 minutes until golden and firm.

The tart is delicious eaten hot with soured cream or yoghurt, but it's also good cold.

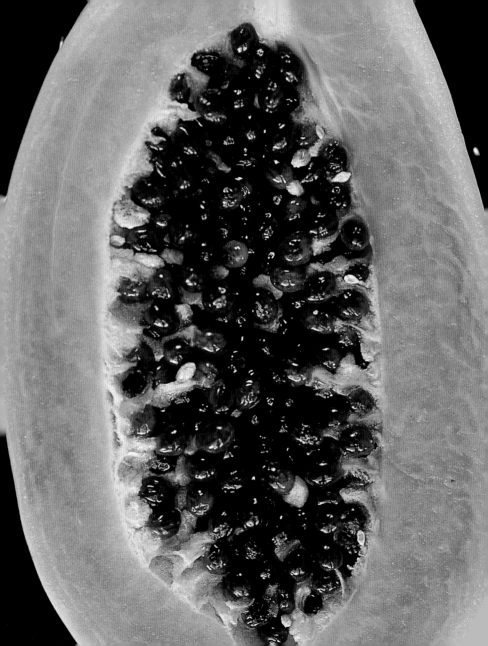

papaya

This fruit is also known as paw paw, or *fruta bomba* to polite Cubans because 'papaya' is slang in their country for the female sexual organs! The buttery soft flesh is most often eaten when it is ripe and orange-coloured, but it is also popular in savoury meals when unripe, hard and green, as in one of my favourite dishes in the world, Thai som tam (page 282). Even the peppery, bitter seeds can be eaten and are said to help get rid of worms. Papaya, particularly when unripe, is a wonderful digestive aid because of a powerful enzyme called papain, which helps break down proteins. The fruit is very soothing for the gut, helping to reduce inflammation and encouraging the elimination of gas and waste products. This is partly because of its rich fibre content, which also helps balance good bacteria in the gut and control cholesterol levels. The papain is also useful in helping calm inflammation elsewhere in the body, such as in the joints. As its colour suggests, papaya is full of beta carotene, as well as vitamin C.

papaya & prawn salad

I FIRST MADE THIS WHEN I WAS LIVING IN BANGKOK, WHERE DELICIOUSLY FRESH
PAPAYAS WERE ABUNDANT AND INEXPENSIVE, BUT COTTAGE CHEESE WAS A RARITY!

2 ripe **papayas**
200g cottage cheese
200g cooked shelled prawns
4 spring **onions**, trimmed
   and finely sliced
juice of 1 **lime**
2 tsp tamari or soy sauce
2 tsp **sesame seeds**

Cut the papayas in half and scoop out the seeds.
In a bowl, roughly mix together the cottage
cheese, prawns, spring onions, lime juice and
tamari, using a fork. Pile the mixture into the
papaya cavities, sprinkle with the sesame seeds
and eat straight away.

griddled papaya with lime honey

ANOTHER CONCOCTION INSPIRED BY MY DAYS IN BANGKOK, WHERE YOU COME ACROSS STREET-HAWKERS SELLING PEELED SLICES OF PAPAYA SPRINKLED WITH LIME JUICE — A SUBLIME FUSION. YOU WILL PROBABLY NEED TO GRIDDLE THE PAPAYA SLICES IN TWO OR THREE BATCHES.

*juice of 2 **limes***
*2 tsp **honey***
*1cm piece fresh root **ginger**, grated*
*2 **papayas**, peeled and sliced*

Preheat a griddle pan. In a bowl, mix together the lime juice, honey and ginger. Swish the papaya slices around in the mixture and then lay them in the hot griddle pan. Cook the papaya slices for about 2 minutes each side, brushing them with the marinade. Serve them hot, as they are or with natural yoghurt.

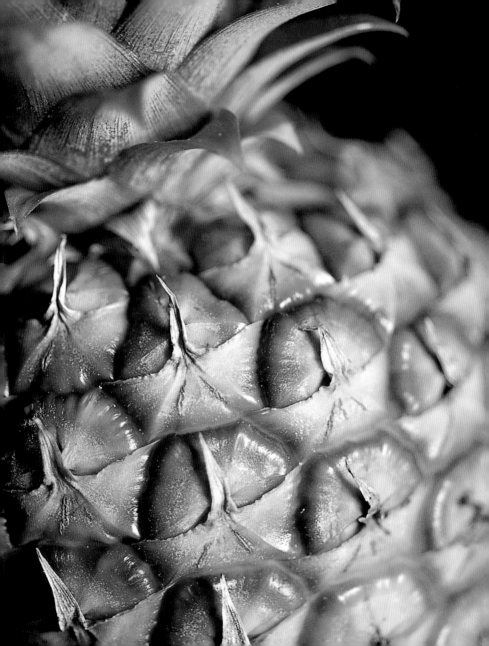

pineapple

Pineapples were so esteemed in 18th century Europe that they were used as prestigious table decorations and to this day, their sweet taste of the tropics is highly prized. A pineapple is actually a collection of flowers, each with its own 'eye', fused around a central core. Fresh pineapple is rich in an enzyme called bromelain that not only helps digestion but can also reduce inflammation. Eaten with a meal, pineapple helps the breakdown of proteins. It is so efficient at this that it is used as a meat tenderiser. For its anti-inflammatory effects, papaya is best eaten between meals; this way it can help relieve the swelling linked to arthritis and sore throats, as well as injuries or operations. Bromelain appears to thin mucus, so it's useful for helping bronchitis, asthma and sinus problems. It also helps reduce the stickiness of blood, and has been shown to relieve angina and thrombosis. Pineapple's high water content, combined with various acids it contains, gives it a diuretic action, which means it can be helpful for high blood pressure.

pineapple fish curry

LIGHT FISH AND TANGY FRESH PINEAPPLE CONTRAST THE RICH COCONUT IN THIS
DELICIOUS CURRY. IF YOU CAN'T FIND KAFFIR LIME LEAVES, JUST LEAVE THEM OUT.

200g chunky **fish**, such as
    monkfish, skinned
2 tsp olive oil
1 medium **onion**, peeled
    and finely diced
2–3cm piece fresh root
    ginger, peeled and
    grated
1 lemongrass stalk, sliced
2 kaffir lime leaves, sliced
3 tbsp Thai red curry paste
1/2 fresh **pineapple**, peeled,
    cored and cubed
600ml **coconut** milk
12–15 **basil** leaves
6–8 coriander sprigs, leaves
    stripped and torn

Cut the fish into bite-sized chunks and set aside.
Heat the olive oil in a large saucepan and cook the
onion with the ginger, lemongrass and kaffir lime
leaves, stirring, for 3–4 minutes until the onion is
soft. Add the Thai curry paste and stir for a couple
of minutes.

Put the fish in the pan and toss gently for a
few minutes to lightly sear the pieces on the
outside, then add the pineapple. Pour in the
coconut milk and leave to cook gently for about
15 minutes.

Just before serving, stir in the basil and torn
coriander leaves. Serve with brown rice.

baked parma ham & chicory rolls

THIS MAKES A GOOD STARTER. THE COMBINATION OF FLAVOURS — BITTER, SWEET
AND SALTY — OFFSET EACH OTHER BRILLIANTLY.

4 heads of chicory (Belgian
    endive)
16 **basil** leaves
½ small **pineapple**, peeled,
    cored and chopped
freshly ground black pepper
8 slices of Parma ham (or
    Serrano)
1 tbsp balsamic vinegar
25g Parmesan cheese,
    freshly grated

Preheat the oven to 180°C/Gas 4. Slice the chicory
in half lengthways and lay two basil leaves and
three or four pieces of pineapple on each half.
Grind a little black pepper over them and wrap
each firmly in a slice of Parma ham.

Lay the rolls in an ovenproof dish and pour in
a little water, enough to just cover the bottom of
the dish. Cover with foil and bake for 20 minutes.

Remove the foil, sprinkle the balsamic vinegar
over the rolls, then scatter over the Parmesan.
Bake for a further 10 minutes or so until the
cheese has melted and the chicory is soft.

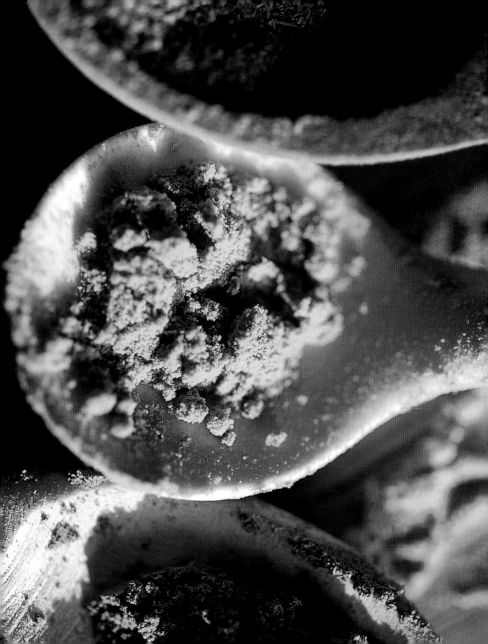

spices

Given their amazing aromas, tastes and health benefits, it's no surprise that wars were fought over spices in past centuries. One of my favourite flavours ever is that of cardamom, which is wonderful in both sweet and savoury dishes. Herbalists recommend it, as well as cinnamon, turmeric and cloves, for their gut soothing properties, which help expel wind, quell nausea and calm gripey pains. Cinnamon is also renowned for its ability to relieve colds, arthritis and high blood pressure. Turmeric, a root related to ginger, is often called 'poor man's saffron' due to its colour, but it is an outstanding spice in its own right. It contains curcumin, which has been widely researched for its abilities to help liver function, and as a powerful anti-inflammatory, it is useful in cases of arthritis, Crohn's disease and ulcerative colitis. Curcumin has even been shown to help protect against cancer. Cloves were an ancient remedy for toothache and apart from pain relief, they are used to ease the symptoms of coughs and colds.

apple rice pudding

OK, SO THIS ISN'T LOADED WITH SUGAR AND CREAM LIKE THE REAL THING, BUT
TRY IT AND YOU'LL SEE HOW GOOD IT IS. FOR A RICE PUDDING IT'S RELATIVELY
QUICK, BECAUSE YOU START OFF COOKING THE RICE ON THE HOB — IN FACT, IT
IS GREAT FOR USING UP LEFTOVER RICE.

150g **brown rice**
10 **cardamom** pods
1 **cinnamon** stick
350ml milk or **soya** milk
1 tbsp sugar or alternative
    equivalent (see page 10)
1 tbsp raisins
¹/₂ **apple**, peeled, cored and
    grated
1 vanilla pod
1 tsp butter
blueberries or **strawberries**,
    to serve

Cook the rice as instructed on the packet, together
with the cardamom pods and cinnamon stick. In
the meantime, preheat the oven to 180°C/Gas 4.
Drain the rice if necessary.

Heat the milk in a saucepan and stir in the
rice, sugar, raisins, grated apple, vanilla pod and
butter. Tip the mixture into a small baking dish
and stir well. Bake for 30 minutes.

Serve with fresh berries and, if you really want
to splash out, some cream.

spicy masala tea

THIS COMPLETE BLEND OF DELICIOUS SPICES MAKES A WARMING, WINTER TEA.
YOU COULD ADD A LITTLE HONEY AS A SWEETENER IF YOU LIKE.

*1cm piece fresh root **ginger**, peeled and finely sliced*
*6 **cardamom** pods*
*1 **cinnamon** stick*
*5 **cloves***
500ml water

Put all the ingredients in a large saucepan and bring to the boil. Lower the heat and leave to simmer for at least 10 minutes. Strain and serve.

NOTE You can leave the pan on the hob and reheat the tea later when you fancy another cup or even over a couple of days, topping up with water and perhaps a few extra spices. The flavour of the cardamom in particular is more pronounced the following day.

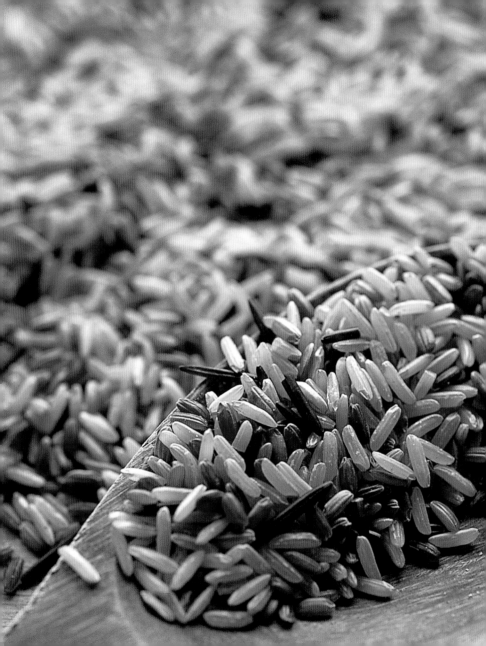

brown rice

Brown rice is slowly losing its reputation as worthy 'hippy food' as more people appreciate its taste and texture, not to mention the nutrient value. It is simply the whole rice grain that has had only the outer hull removed. The process that transforms brown rice into white rice removes most of the vitamin stores, at least half of the minerals, all of the dietary fibre and all of the essential fatty acids. Fibre is best known for encouraging healthy bowel movements; in keeping the elimination of wastes regular, you minimise your risk of problems such as diverticulitis and even colon cancer. Fibre also slows down the release of the starch as sugar into the bloodstream, making for a more satisfying meal and a steady release of energy. Rice is a naturally gluten-free starch, important for people who cannot digest gluten grains such as wheat and oats. Many people make the mistake of not cooking brown rice for long enough so it ends up *al dente* rather than slightly chewy.

mushroom risotto

THIS IS A REMARKABLY 'CLEAN-FEELING' RISOTTO COMPARED WITH THE HEAVIER VERSIONS MADE WITH CREAM. IT'S GREAT AS A MAIN COURSE SERVED WITH A WONDERFOODS GREEN SALAD (PAGE 111). MISO IS A JAPANESE-STYLE SOYA BEAN PASTE SOLD IN MOST HEALTH FOOD SHOPS AND MANY SUPERMARKETS.

3 tbsp miso (**soya** paste)
3 mugfuls of water
1 mugful of white wine
1 tbsp dried **seaweed**, such as arame
4 **shallots**, peeled and finely diced
2 **garlic** cloves, peeled and crushed
1 tbsp olive oil
200g shiitake **mushrooms**, sliced
1cm piece fresh root **ginger**, peeled and finely sliced
1 red chilli, deseeded and sliced
1 mugful of **brown rice**
1 tbsp torn coriander leaves

In one saucepan, mix the miso with the water and wine, add the seaweed and bring to a simmer.

In another pan, soften the shallots and garlic in the olive oil until translucent, then add the mushrooms, ginger and chilli. Stir for a few minutes before adding the rice.

Turn up the heat under the miso mixture to bring it to the boil, then add it to the rice. Stir and cover with the lid. Turn down to the lowest setting and leave to cook gently for 40 minutes.

To serve, pile the risotto on to plates and top with a sprinkling of coriander leaves.

scented savoury rice

THIS IS A WONDERFULLY AROMATIC WAY OF COOKING RICE, ESPECIALLY TO ACCOMPANY A DISH SUCH AS MOROCCAN LAMB (PAGE 194). TO GET THE RIGHT RATIO OF WATER TO RICE I FIND IT EASIEST TO MEASURE BOTH BY VOLUME, USING A MUG, RATHER THAN WEIGHING THE RICE.

1 mugful of **brown rice**
2¹/₂ mugfuls of water
6 **cardamom** pods
4 **cloves**
¹/₂ **cinnamon** stick
¹/₂ tsp ground **turmeric**

Put all the ingredients in a large saucepan and bring to the boil. Cover with a lid and turn the heat down to a simmer. Cook until the rice is soft and chewy rather than al dente; this should take about 40 minutes. (I usually cheat and use an electric rice cooker which gets the water evaporation right every time.)

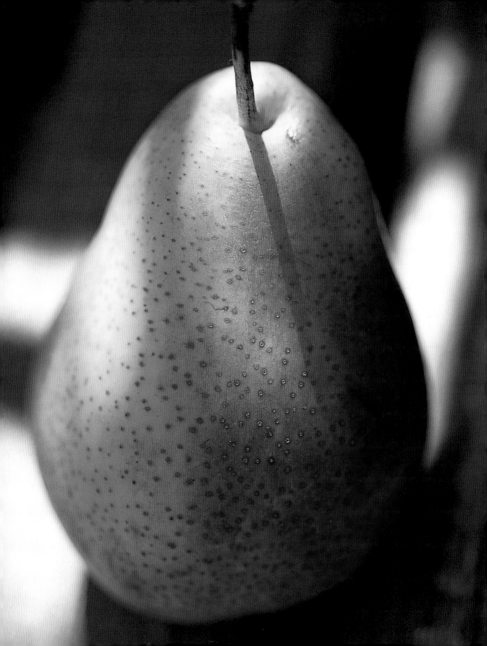

pear

When you bite into a ripe pear and the juice dribbles down your arm, you can see why Homer referred to this fruit as a 'gift of the gods'. Pears have much in common with their distant relative, the apple: many shapes, sizes, hues and health benefits. Pears are higher in the soluble fibre pectin than apples, which make them very cleansing and soothing for the whole digestive tract. Not only does pectin help keep the bowels moving well, it also binds to waste products and cancer-causing substances in the colon. When ripe, pears are very easy to break down, which makes them gentle on the digestion and a good source of energy that, combined with the fibre, releases only gradually. Pears are generally considered one of the foods least likely to trigger an allergic reaction so they are an ideal fruit to introduce to babies being weaned and anyone with a sensitive system. Unlike many fruits, pears are best ripened after picking, so they turn buttery and don't develop a grainy texture.

pear & feta salad

MY PREFERRED VARIETY OF PEAR IS WILLIAMS BUT YOU CAN USE ANY TYPE YOU
LIKE. AND YOU CAN EXCHANGE THE FETA FOR GOAT'S CHEESE OR EVEN A GOOD
BLUE CHEESE.

2 ripe but firm **pears**
150g feta cheese
150g **spinach**, washed
100g rocket, washed
50g shelled **walnuts**
2 tsp balsamic vinegar
1 tbsp **walnut** oil

Quarter the pears lengthways, remove the cores
and then cut into eighths. Cut the feta cheese into
eight slices.

Toss the spinach, rocket and walnuts with the
balsamic vinegar and walnut oil and pile on to
four plates. Arrange the pear and feta slices on top
and serve.

morning zing juice

THE TASTE AND TEXTURE OF MELON JUICE SOMEHOW CONJURE UP THE SENSATION
OF CREAMINESS, ALL OFFSET BY THE SHARP GINGER AND SWEET MINT.

3 ripe but firm **pears**
1 thick slice of **melon**,
peeled and deseeded
1cm piece fresh root **ginger**,
peeled
small bunch of mint

Chop the pears and melon into pieces small
enough to fit through the opening of your juicer.
Push all the ingredients through, one by one and
drink the juice straight away. Well, once you've
washed up the juicer perhaps!

NOTE If you don't own a juicer, you can make a
smoothie using a blender, but you will need to use
slightly over-ripe pears. Peel, core and chop the
pears, chop the melon and grate the ginger. Whiz
in a blender with the mint until liquidised, then
thin with a little water if necessary.

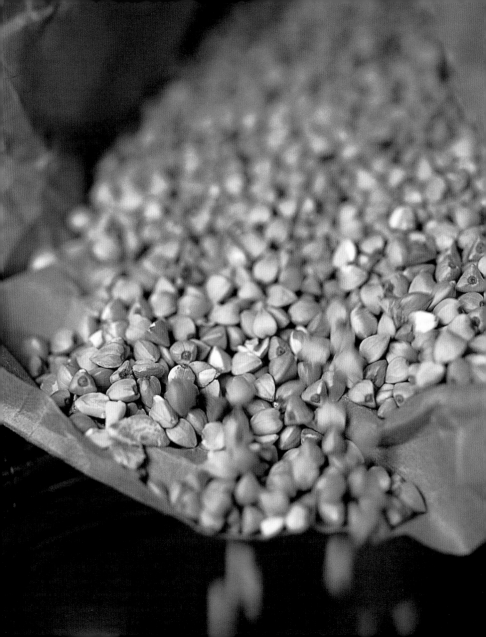

buckwheat

Buckwheat was introduced to Europe by the Crusaders and later the Turks, which is how it got its original name 'Saracen wheat'. Contrary to the name, buckwheat isn't a grain, but a fruit seed related to rhubarb. This makes it a good alternative for anyone avoiding the gluten grains (wheat, oats, rye and barley), including people who find gluten triggers digestive problems or depression. Buckwheat contains fibre and all eight essential amino acids, so, for a grain-like food, it is a good source of protein. Although it's not particularly high in the amino acid tryptophan, the carb content means there's more chance of the tryptophan being converted to serotonin, which boosts moods. The rich magnesium in buckwheat is useful for relaxing the nervous system and muscles – including those in the bowel, which can alleviate constipation. Buckwheat is notably rich in an antioxidant called rutin that helps to strengthen blood capillaries and prevent the platelets in the blood from clotting together.

buckwheat crêpes

100g **buckwheat** flour
pinch of salt
1 **egg**
150ml milk or **soya** milk
150ml water
splash of olive oil

Put the flour and salt in a mixing bowl, make a well in the middle and add the egg. Mix the milk and water together in a jug. Beat the egg into the flour, adding a little of the liquid at a time, plus a splash of olive oil, to make a smooth batter. Ideally, leave the batter to stand for at least 1 hour.

When you're ready to cook the crêpes, lightly oil a frying pan and heat it well. Pour in about 1 tbsp batter and tilt the pan around to spread the batter to the edge. Cook for 1–2 minutes until the crêpe is golden underneath, then flip it over and cook the other side for a minute or so. Remove and stack the crêpes on a warm plate, separating them with greaseproof paper; keep warm. Repeat with the rest of the batter.

Serve the crêpes with your choice of topping, sweet or savoury.

soba noodles & salmon

SOBA ARE JAPANESE NOODLES MADE USING BUCKWHEAT FLOUR. THEY HAVE A VERY DISTINCT FLAVOUR.

*300g dried soba (**buckwheat**) noodles*
*grated zest of 1 **lime***
*juice of 2 **limes***
1 small chilli, deseeded and sliced
1 tbsp brown sugar
1 tsp ground coriander
1 tbsp tamari or soy sauce
*4 small **salmon** fillets*
splash of olive oil
*4 **shallots**, peeled and finely diced*
*1 tbsp **sesame** oil*
2 tbsp chopped coriander leaves

Cook the soba noodles in a pan of boiling water for 6–8 minutes until *al dente*. Drain, rinse in cold water and drain the noodles well.

In a bowl, mix together the lime zest and juice, chilli, sugar, ground coriander and tamari. Add the salmon fillets and turn to coat them in the mixture; set aside.

Heat a wok, add a splash of olive oil and soften the shallots until translucent. Add the salmon fillets together with the marinade and cook for about 2–3 minutes each side, or until cooked to your taste – you could just sear them briefly. Remove the fish and set aside.

Add the noodles to the wok with the sesame oil and toss to heat them through. Divide the noodles among four plates, lay a piece of salmon on each pile and scatter with the coriander.

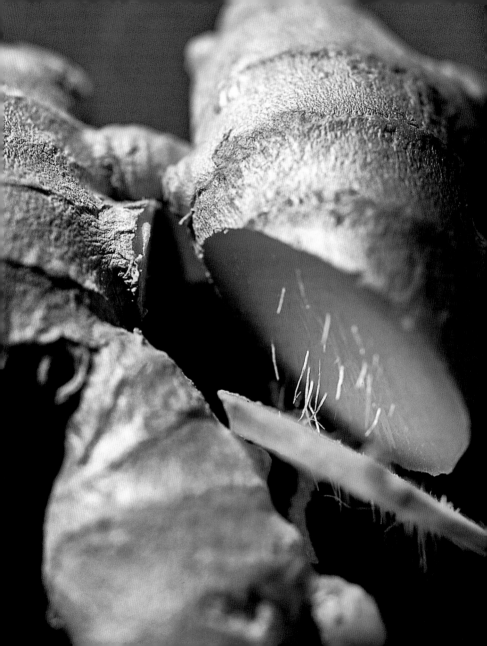

ginger

Ginger has been used for centuries as a medicinal and spiritual cleanser. In Ayurvedic and traditional Chinese medicine, it occurs in half of all prescriptions. The versatility of this hot, refreshing, juicy root makes it a good addition to both sweet and savoury dishes, as well as to a medicine cabinet. Ginger's primary health uses are in calming the gut – it not only helps to quell nausea but also to soothe gripes, diarrhoea and wind. Studies have suggested that it also has a role in preventing motion sickness and vomiting in pregnancy, as well as the ability to help ulcers heal. Several natural chemicals in ginger, including gingerols, inhibit inflammatory substances in the body, making it particularly useful for anyone with arthritis, asthma or other conditions involving inflammation. On the cardiovascular front, ginger reduces the stickiness of blood, tones the heart and reduces cholesterol levels. As well as for digestive upsets and respiratory tract infections, Western herbalists also recommend ginger as a stimulant that warms the body and boosts circulation.

baked gingered fish

YOU CAN USE ANY WHITE FISH FOR THIS DISH, BUT MY FAVOURITE IS THE
DELICIOUS, RICH ANTARCTIC ICEFISH, WHICH IS AVAILABLE FROM MANY
FISHMONGERS AND SOME SUPERMARKET FRESH FISH COUNTERS.

*4 white **fish** steaks*
4 tbsp water
FOR THE MARINADE
2–3cm piece fresh root
  ***ginger**, peeled and*
  grated
*2 **garlic** cloves, peeled and*
  crushed
grated zest and juice of
  *1 **lime***
2 tsp tamari or soy sauce
1 red chilli, deseeded and
  sliced

Combine all the ingredients for the marinade in a shallow ovenproof dish. Add the fish steaks and turn to coat them in the mixture. Ideally, set aside to marinate for 2 or 3 hours, but if you haven't got that long you'll find the dish still tastes great.

Preheat the oven to 200°C/Gas 6. Add the water to the marinade in the dish and stir it in well. Bake for 15–20 minutes or until the fish steaks are cooked through. Icefish usually takes a little longer than most other white fish because the texture is quite dense.

Eat with stir-fried vegetables and a little brown rice or Herby sweet oven chips (page 198).

roasted pears with lime & ginger

THIS EASY-TO-PREPARE DESSERT WILL KEEP IN THE FRIDGE FOR A COUPLE OF DAYS — YOU MIGHT EVEN BE TEMPTED TO HAVE SOME FOR BREAKFAST. THE PEARS CAN BE CUT UP AND COOKED IN THE PAN WITH THE SYRUP IF YOU LIKE, TO MAKE A SORT OF COMPOTE.

200ml water
2.5cm piece fresh root **ginger**, peeled and finely sliced
1 tbsp **honey**
grated zest and juice of 1 **lime**
100ml white wine
4 ripe but firm **pears**
TO SERVE
6 tbsp natural **yoghurt**
$^1/_2$ tsp ground **cinnamon**
$^1/_2$ tsp vanilla extract
4 mint leaves (optional)

Preheat the oven to 180°C/Gas 4. Put the water, ginger, honey, lime juice and zest in a saucepan. Bring to the boil, then add the wine. Leave to simmer for 10 minutes.

Meanwhile, quarter and core the pears and lay them in an ovenproof dish. Pour the ginger and lime mixture over the pears and bake them for about 30 minutes.

Meanwhile, mix the yoghurt with the cinnamon and vanilla extract. When the pears are tender, place two halves on each plate. Top with a dollop of the flavoured yoghurt, and if you're feeling fancy finish with a mint leaf.

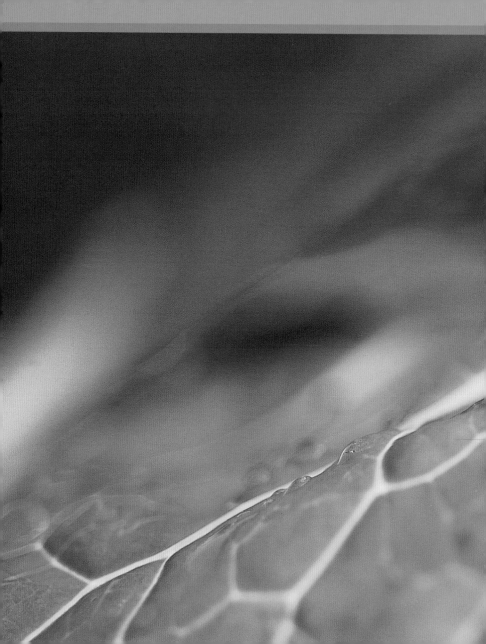

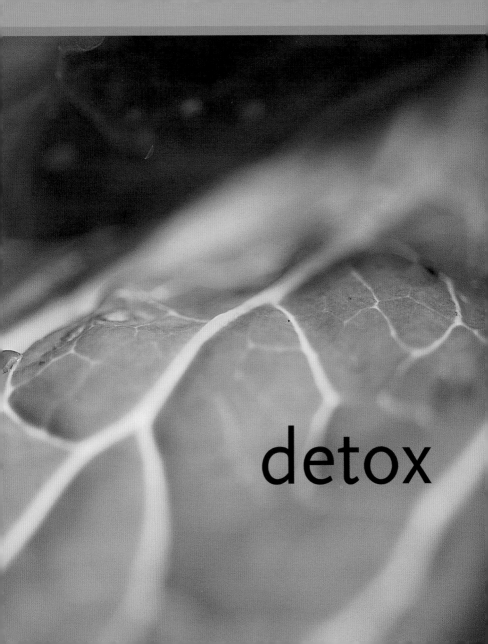

detox

Detoxing has become something of a buzz word in the last few years and countless books have been published on detox programmes. This is not what this section of Wonderfoods is about! The foods here are ones that contain nutrients which enhance the body's natural, ongoing, normal detoxification processes. It's easy to forget, with the books and magazine articles on detoxing, that it is something our bodies do permanently – every hour of every day. The wonderfoods here can help to optimise that process.

Although all cells do their own housework throughout the body, the liver is the main organ of detoxification. It is best known for processing challenging substances like alcohol, but this vital organ has many roles. Its other important tasks include storing glucose and helping balance blood levels of this crucial fuel, storing other nutrients, breaking down fats, making cholesterol, forming proteins and producing bile salts to help with digestion.

So making sure the liver is in good shape is vital for health. If this key organ is being overwhelmed, you're likely to feel tired, sluggish, achey and have poor digestion or bad skin. All the wonderfoods in this section are rich in antioxidant nutrients, which the liver needs in high doses. From humble vitamin C to the glucosinolates in broccoli and kale, a spectrum of antioxidants keeps the liver ticking over well. Another nutrient required for detoxification in the liver is sulphur. It is generally recognised that a common reason for feeling run down and sluggish is exceeding your body's capacity to detoxify what you put in it.

To keep your detox processes working efficiently you need to load up on the foods that are good for your liver, such as the wonderfoods in this section, and minimise your intake of foods and other substances that tax it. So cutting back on alcohol, caffeine, fatty foods, salty foods, processed sugars and food additives lessens the burden on your body's detox capacity. Even before 'detox diet' became trendy, many cultures had for hundreds of years valued periods of abstention of such substances for both spiritual and health reasons and we would do well to follow suit.

Many people find that lightening the load on their liver and boosting it with selected foods such as the detox wonderfoods makes them feel energised, alert and clearer in both their mind and body.

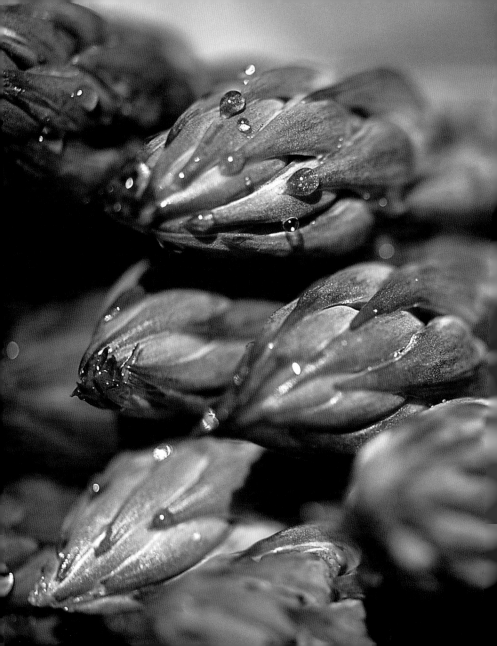

asparagus

Asparagus was cultivated in all corners of the Roman empire and was known as 'sparrowgrass' in Britain in the 18th century. Not only is it still a delicacy, this vegetable is loaded with goodness. In one serving, you get two-thirds of your daily need for folic acid, which is not only crucial for the proper development of a baby but also good heart health. Asparagus also contains an amino acid called asparagine. This, along with its high potassium content and low sodium, makes it a diuretic and cleanser, useful for processing proteins and flushing through the kidneys. Diuretics not only help reduce blood pressure but also water retention in the legs and premenstrually. Asparagus is a source of the flavonoid, rutin, which has an affinity for healthy blood capillaries, helping prevent them from rupturing, such as in haemorrhoids. Because of its phallic shape, asparagus was considered to be an aphrodisiac but unfortunately, it doesn't actually seem to have any chemical properties that would hold that true.

griddled asparagus with serrano ham

THE FINER THE ASPARAGUS SPEARS, THE MORE TENDER AND SWEET THEY ARE. IF YOU CAN GET HOLD OF THEM, THE SPANISH WHITE ASPARAGUS MAKE THIS DISH A REAL DELICACY.

splash of olive oil
1 tbsp balsamic vinegar
16–20 **asparagus** spears
8 slices of Serrano ham (or Parma)

Heat a splash of olive oil and the balsamic vinegar in a well-seasoned griddle pan or non-stick frying pan. When it's hot, add the asparagus spears and cook until lightly charred on one side. Turn and cook them on the other side until they are just limp. Arrange the griddled asparagus on plates with the slices of Serrano ham and serve.

asparagus chicken stir-fry

BECAUSE ASPARAGUS AND CHICKEN BOTH HAVE QUITE DELICATE FLAVOURS,
NEITHER CROWDS THE OTHER OUT IN THIS LIGHT MEAL.

a little sesame oil
*2 **shallots**, peeled and finely diced*
*1 **garlic** clove, peeled and crushed*
¹/₂ tsp Chinese five spice powder
*2 large **chicken** breasts, skinned and sliced*
*12 thin **asparagus** spears, trimmed and sliced*
2 tbsp water
2 tsp tamari or soy sauce
*2 tsp **sesame seeds***

Heat a wok and add a little sesame oil, then add the shallots and garlic with the five spice powder and sauté until softened. Add the chicken slices and toss over the heat for a few minutes until the chicken is nearly cooked through.

Add the asparagus, water and tamari, toss well, then cover and cook for a couple of minutes until the asparagus and chicken are cooked.

Serve the stir-fry sprinkled with sesame seeds, on a bed of rice noodles.

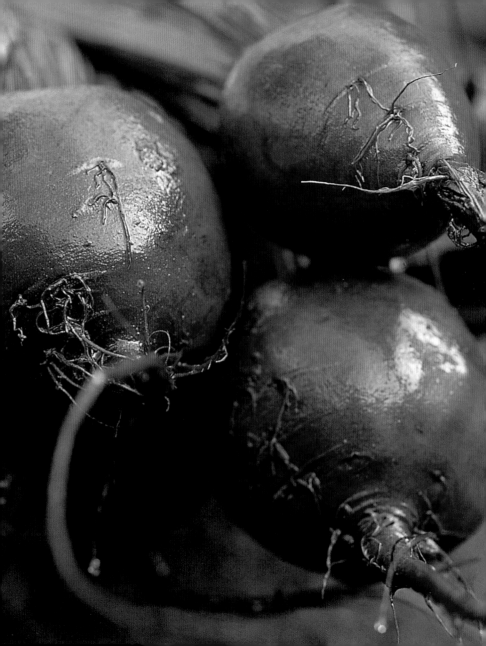

beetroot

Stunningly coloured beetroot are loaded with nutrients and, as their hues suggest, are considered very purifying for the blood. They have been used over the centuries as folk remedies for anaemia, menstrual problems and kidney disorders, and now modern science is revealing their wonders. One constituent of this root vegetable that contributes to their deep red colour is betacyanin. This and other powerful antioxidants in beetroot have been shown to enhance detoxing processes in the liver and even help protect against cancer of the skin, lungs and colon. Studies have indicated that beetroot extracts increase the activity of the body's natural antioxidant enzymes in the liver, such as glutathione peroxidase. Beetroot has also been shown to help lower cholesterol and increase the ratio of the HDL 'good cholesterol' to the LDL 'bad' type. In addition to the roots, beet tops (or leaves) are highly nutritious – loaded with iron and beta carotene. Beetroot is most commonly eaten boiled, but it is wonderful roasted – and eaten raw, particularly if it's grated.

marinated red onion & beetroot salad

IF YOU'RE NOT USED TO HAVING RAW BEETROOT, THIS IS A GOOD RECIPE TO START WITH. YOU CAN EXCHANGE THE FETA FOR A GOOD GOAT'S CHEESE IF YOU LIKE.

2 medium **beetroot**, peeled and grated
$\frac{1}{2}$ red **onion**, peeled and very finely sliced
juice of 1$\frac{1}{2}$ **lemons**
1 tbsp olive oil
1 tbsp chopped **parsley**
fine sea salt
2 handfuls of **watercress**, trimmed
150g feta cheese, crumbled

In a bowl, toss the grated beetroot and slivers of red onion with the lemon juice. Leave to marinate, ideally overnight.

Just before serving, mix in the olive oil and chopped parsley and season with a little sea salt.

Arrange the watercress on plates, spoon on the beetroot mixture and top with crumbled feta. Serve with hot rye bread.

roasted beetroot soup

THIS VIVID SOUP IS EQUALLY GOOD HOT OR COLD. A SWIRL OF NATURAL YOGHURT IS THE PERFECT CONTRAST.

1kg **beetroot**, peeled and
   chopped
1 large **onion**, cut into
   8 wedges (unpeeled)
2 tsp caraway seeds
4–6 **thyme** sprigs
freshly ground black pepper
olive oil, to drizzle
700ml chicken or vegetable
   stock
juice of ½ **lemon**
TO SERVE
natural **yoghurt**
2 tbsp chopped **parsley**

Preheat the oven to 180°C/Gas 4. Put the beetroot and onion pieces in a roasting tray with the caraway seeds and thyme. Season with pepper, drizzle with olive oil and toss well. Roast in the oven for 30–40 minutes until the beetroot feels tender when pierced with a skewer.

Remove the papery skin from the onion, then tip the contents of the tray into a large saucepan. Add the stock and lemon juice and heat gently to a simmer. Take off the heat and whiz to a smooth consistency using a hand-held stick blender (or use a free-standing blender, then reheat gently to serve hot).

As you serve the soup, top each portion with a spoonful of yoghurt and swirl decoratively. Sprinkle with the chopped parsley.

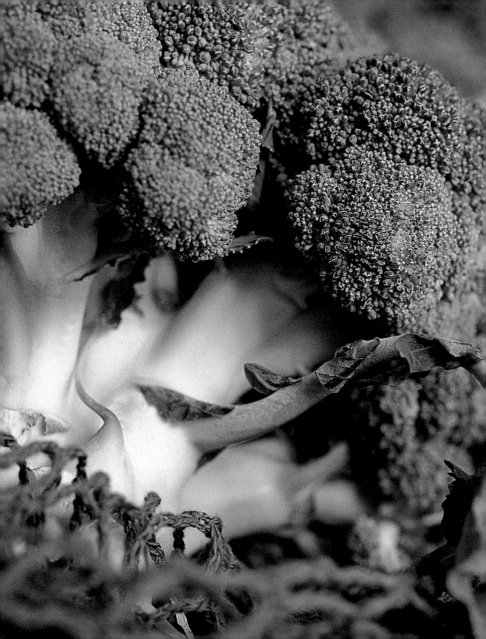

broccoli & kale

Broccoli and kale are just two of the cruciferous family, so called because of the cross-like structure of their stems. Brussels sprouts, cabbage, cauliflower and purple-sprouting broccoli are cousins. Kale and broccoli in particular are two of the most power-packed veg! Broccoli is rich in vitamin C and kale is one of the highest antioxidant foods there is. Both are excellent sources of fibre, which helps keep the bowel working efficiently and feeds good bacteria there. Broccoli and kale are also rich sources of glucosinolates, which have powerful actions in the detoxification processes in the liver. Of these, sulforaphane, sinigrin and indole-3-carbinol (I3C), have been found to be power anti-cancer substances. I3C is involved in processing oestrogen, helping balance menstrual cycles and potentially protecting against breast cancer. Both, but kale in particular, are loaded with beta carotene and its relatives, lutein and zeaxanthin. These chemicals are good for immunity, but especially for protecting the eye against sunlight damage and age-related macular degeneration.

broccoli & sweet potato salad

THIS WONDERFUL COMBINATION FIRST PAST MY LIPS IN A CAFE IN AUCKLAND AND IT'S BEEN A FIRM LUNCH FAVOURITE IN OUR HOUSE EVER SINCE.

2 **sweet potatoes**, scrubbed and cut into 1cm discs
1 **red pepper**, cored, deseeded and sliced
3–4 **thyme** sprigs
olive oil, to drizzle
1 head of **broccoli**, cut into florets
150g feta cheese, cubed
1 tbsp **sunflower seeds**
1 tbsp cider vinegar
freshly ground black pepper

Preheat the oven to 180°C/Gas 4. Put the sweet potatoes, red pepper and thyme sprigs in a roasting tray and drizzle with some olive oil. Toss well and roast in the oven for about 30 minutes until the potatoes are tender. Set aside to cool.

Meanwhile, plunge the broccoli florets into a pan of boiling water and blanch for no more than a minute. Drain and refresh in cold water, then drain thoroughly.

When all the vegetables are cool, toss them in a bowl with the feta, sunflower seeds, cider vinegar, pepper to taste and a little more olive oil. Serve at once.

green spice stir-fry

IF I'M COOKING A FISH OR MEAT CURRY, I FIND THIS IS A GOOD, LIGHT SIDE DISH
TO SERVE ALONGSIDE, RATHER THAN JUST ANOTHER SAUCY CURRY.

1 tsp cumin seeds
1 tbsp olive oil
1 **garlic** clove, peeled and
    crushed
1 small chilli, deseeded
    and sliced
1 head of **broccoli**, cut into
    florets
8–10 **kale** leaves, torn off
    the stalks
2 tbsp water

Toast the cumin seeds in a dry wok over a medium heat until they are lightly browned and giving off a lovely aroma. Add the olive oil, garlic and chilli and stir for a minute or two, then add the broccoli, kale and water. Stir over the heat for a few minutes until the kale leaves are wilted and the broccoli is cooked through but still slightly crunchy.

Serve at once, with brown rice and Moroccan lamb (page 194) or Pineapple fish curry (page 58).

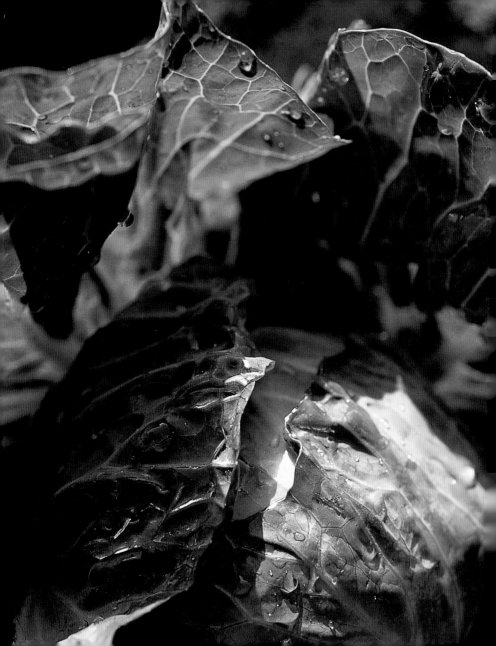

cabbage

The humble, common cabbage may not be the classiest of vegetables but it is one of the richest, healthwise. Even ancient Egyptians knew how good it was for the liver – apparently they ate loads in advance of drinking binges! Like its relatives broccoli and kale, cabbage contains a range of powerful, sulphurous substances that protect the liver, boost its detox capacity, aid the processing of hormones and can even help protect against certain cancers. Sulphur, sometimes referred to as the 'beauty mineral', is also needed for healthy skin, hair and nails. Cabbage juice, although hardly a gastronomic delight, is a traditional remedy for peptic ulcers. In addition to their high fibre content, cabbages are packed with nutrients such as vitamin C, folic acid, calcium, potassium and many more. Cabbage that is overcooked and soggy is unpalatable, but lightly blanched or stir-fried, or even shredded raw in salads it's delicious. Red cabbage has even more goodness than white or green, plus a striking touch of colour.

keralan cabbage

WHILE BEING PUNTED ALONG THE TRANQUIL BACKWATERS OF KERALA IN
SOUTHERN INDIA, I FEASTED ON LOCAL DISHES PREPARED BY THOMAS THE CHEF,
INCLUDING THIS ONE. YOU CAN BUY CURRY LEAVES, FRESH OR DRIED, FROM ASIAN
GROCERS AND SOME SUPERMARKETS.

1 tbsp **coconut** oil (or
  olive oil)
1 tsp mustard seeds
1 tbsp curry leaves
1 green chilli, deseeded
  and finely sliced
1 tsp cumin seeds
1/2 tsp ground **turmeric**
1cm piece fresh root,
  ginger, peeled and
  grated
2 tbsp grated **coconut**
  (ideally fresh, otherwise
  use dried)
1 **onion**, peeled and very
  finely diced
1/3 **cabbage**, very finely
  shredded

Heat a wok and add the oil (ideally coconut).
Throw in the mustard seeds, curry leaves, chilli,
cumin seeds, turmeric and ginger, and stir for a
minute or two. Add the coconut and onion and
cook, stirring, for 3–4 minutes.

Add the cabbage to the spice mixture and stir
and toss for about 5 minutes. Serve immediately,
with spicy grilled fish and rice.

salmon rolls

VIETNAMESE SPRING ROLLS AND CHINESE DUCK PANCAKES WERE THE INSPIRATION FOR THESE! OTHER THAN TASTING FANTASTIC, THEY ARE A FUN WAY TO SHARE FOOD AROUND A TABLE WITH FRIENDS.

4 small **salmon** fillets
12 large Savoy **cabbage**
    leaves (at least)
½ **cucumber**, cut into strips
4–6 spring **onions**,
    trimmed and finely
    shredded lengthways
large handful of **bean
    sprouts**
8–10 tbsp tamari or soy
    sauce
2.5cm piece fresh root
    ginger, peeled and
    grated
3 tbsp toasted **sesame** oil

Steam or poach the salmon until just tender, roughly break it up with a fork, then tip it into a serving bowl and leave to cool.

Bring a large saucepan of water to the boil and blanch the cabbage leaves for about 2 minutes until pliable. Drain and refresh under cold water, then drain well and lay on a serving plate.

Arrange the cucumber, spring onions and bean sprouts on another serving plate. Mix the tamari, grated ginger and sesame oil in two small serving bowls or individual dipping bowls.

Put all the serving dishes on the table and let guests help themselves. To eat, you simply roll some salmon and vegetables in a cabbage leaf and dip it into the sauce.

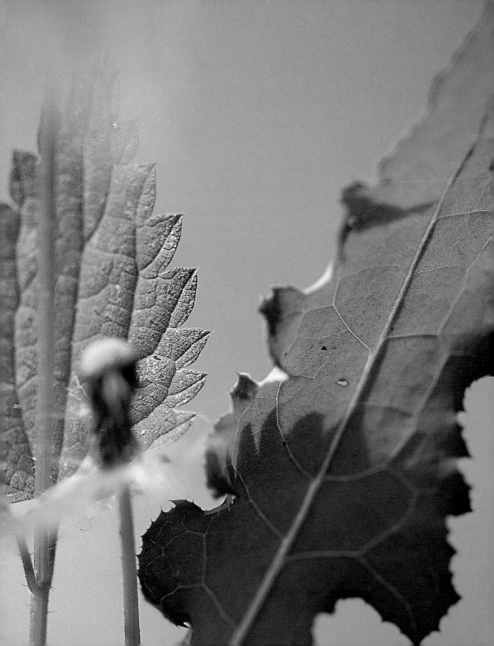

dandelion &
nettles

If you're a gardener you may see these as pernicious weeds and slay them at all costs. Before you do, pick the leaves and make the most of their outstanding properties. Spring is the best time to harvest dandelion, when the leaves are at their most tender and sweet – eat them raw in salads or cooked, like spinach. The roots too are good, eaten raw or stir-fried. Dandelion is considered by herbalists to be one of the best liver tonics; it helps the actual liver detoxification and also the flow of bile to and from the gall bladder. The bitterness of the leaves stimulates digestion, especially of fats, and this, along with their soluble fibre, encourages bowel movements. Dandelion is also useful for combating water retention. As for stinging nettles, don gloves to pick the young shoots at the top of the stems and cook them like spinach. The cooking process destroys the poison that makes them sting and you are left with flavourful greens that have been used for centuries to treat water retention and kidney disorders, and to stimulate the liver and digestion.

warm dandelion & sunchoke salad

ARGAN OIL FROM MOROCCO IS A WONDERFUL NUTTY OIL, RICH IN OMEGA 6 FATS, THAT YOU CAN BUY FROM MOST HEALTH FOOD SHOPS AND SOME SUPERMARKETS.

8 *Jerusalem artichokes*,
    well scrubbed
juice of $1/2$ *lemon*, plus
    a squeeze
1 tbsp *pumpkin* seeds
handful of tender
    dandelion leaves
2 spring *onions*, trimmed
    and sliced
1 tbsp chopped *parsley*
1 tbsp argan oil
pinch of fine sea salt
freshly ground black pepper
150g goat's cheese,
    crumbled

Boil the Jerusalem artichokes (sunchokes) in water to cover, with the juice of $1/2$ lemon added, until they feel tender when pierced with a skewer, about 15 minutes. Drain and allow to cool.

Meanwhile, lightly toast the pumpkin seeds in a dry frying pan.

When the Jerusalem artichokes are cooked and cool, cut them into discs and combine with the dandelion leaves, pumpkin seeds, spring onions and parsley. Drizzle with the argan oil and a squeeze of lemon juice, and season with salt and pepper. Toss to mix and serve topped with the crumbled goat's cheese.

mackerel with nettles

THIS 'EXOTIC' RECIPE COMES FROM DORSET, WHERE MY FRIEND JAMES VERNER FIRST ENCOURAGED ME TO TRY EATING NETTLES. IF YOU CANNOT STEAM THE NETTLES AS THE RECIPE SUGGESTS, RINSE THEM IN WATER AND COOK THEM IN A DRY SAUCEPAN AS YOU WOULD SPINACH. DRINK THE REMAINING LIQUOR, WHICH IS VERY CLEANSING.

5 red chillies
1 **garlic** clove, peeled
handful of **sage, thyme**
     and **parsley** leaves
2 tbsp olive oil
4 **mackerels**, gutted, heads
     on
25 stinging **nettle** tips
dash of balsamic vinegar
4 **lemon** slices

Using a pestle and mortar, pound 1 halved and deseeded chilli with the garlic, herbs and about 1 tbsp olive oil. Stuff the mixture into the fish cavities and secure the opening with a cocktail stick. Preheat the grill.

Steam the nettles until they lose their sting; this takes about 5 minutes.

Meanwhile, cook the mackerel under the hot grill for about 3–4 minutes each side.

Toss the nettles in 1 tbsp olive oil and a dash of balsamic vinegar, then spread them out on plates. Lay a mackerel on each bed of nettles and garnish with a twist of lemon and a whole chilli.

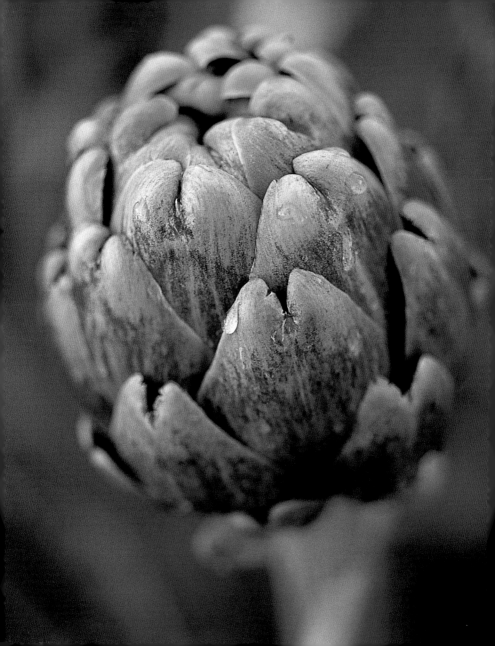

globe artichoke

Surprisingly, perhaps, this vegetable is a member of the thistle family. Medicinally, it is best known for supporting the liver and gall bladder, i.e. it is useful in boosting detoxification and digestion. This is particularly due to natural chemicals it contains, such as cynarin. Recent studies have even shown extracts of artichoke to help relieve the symptoms of irritable bowel syndrome, such as nausea, pain, constipation and wind. It also has antifungal properties. Herbalists recommend globe artichoke for its diuretic properties – helping relieve water retention and high blood pressure. Another bonus for the cardiovascular system is that globe artichoke has been shown to reduce levels of LDL, the so-called 'bad cholesterol'. Antioxidant flavonoids from the artichoke, such as luteolin, help to prevent LDL oxidation, which may reduce the risk of atherosclerosis, or thickening and hardening of the arteries. When you buy globe artichokes, it is the unopened flower heads of the plant that are eaten – choose ones that feel heavy for their size.

stuffed artichokes

'POGGI POGGI' IS THE RIDICULOUS NAME IN OUR FAMILY, COINED BY MY COUSIN
LIZZIE, FOR TRADITIONAL MALTESE STUFFED ARTICHOKES, AS PREPARED BY OUR
GRANDMOTHER AND NOW BY MY AUNTIE MARLENE. THE PROPER MALTESE NAME IS
QAQOCC MIMLI, WHERE THE 'Q' HAS A GLOTTAL STOP SOUND.

*4 large **globe artichokes**, trimmed*
FOR THE STUFFING
6 slices of brown bread, toasted and crumbed
*6 **garlic** cloves, peeled and crushed*
4 anchovy fillets, chopped and mashed
*large handful of flat leaf **parsley**, finely chopped*
*1 tbsp chopped **oregano***
3 tbsp olive oil
freshly ground black pepper
TO SERVE
olive oil
*squeeze of **lemon** juice*

Mix all the stuffing ingredients together in a bowl. Take each artichoke and slam its top on the kitchen counter to open up the leaves. Push generous amounts of stuffing down in between the leaves.

Stand the artichokes in a large saucepan and add enough water to come 2–3cm up their sides. Cover and steam until they are tender, about 40 minutes.

Serve each artichoke on a plate with a side dish of olive oil flavoured with a little lemon juice in which to dip each leaf base as it is pulled. Scrape the flesh and accompanying stuffing off each leaf with your teeth before discarding the rough, hairy choke and enjoying the tender heart.

artichoke heart pizzas

THESE WONDERFUL STARTERS COULD BE MADE IN BULK TO SERVE AS CANAPÉS.
AS YOU'LL SEE, THE 'PIZZA' BASE IS ACTUALLY AN ARTICHOKE HEART. YOU CAN
LEAVE OUT THE ANCHOVIES FOR A VEGETARIAN VERSION.

4 **shallots**, peeled and
   finely diced
1 **garlic** clove, peeled and
   crushed
a little olive oil
8 **artichoke** hearts
1 tsp chopped **parsley**
2 **tomatoes**, sliced
8 **basil** leaves
4 anchovies, cut in half
30g Parmesan cheese,
   freshly grated
8 black olives, stoned
freshly ground black pepper
rocket leaves, to serve

Preheat the oven to 180°C/Gas 4. In a small frying
pan, soften the shallots and garlic in a little olive
oil until translucent.

Lay the artichoke hearts on a baking tray and
spread a little of the cooked shallot mixture on
each, then sprinkle with the parsley. Layer the
tomato slices, basil leaves, anchovies and grated
Parmesan on top. Add an olive, season with
pepper and bake for 15–20 minutes.

Serve as a starter, on a bed of rocket leaves.

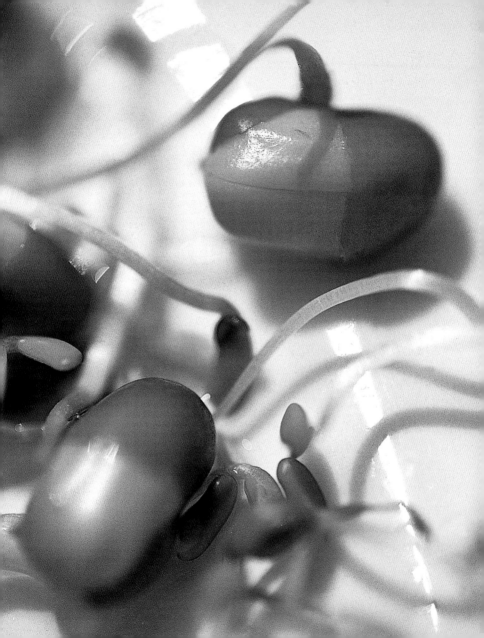

alfalfa &
mung sprouts

Grow your own sprouts from dormant seeds and you can benefit from the concentrated nutrients they offer as they spring to life and become edible. Sprouts contain phyto-nutrients, similar, yet more condensed than those in the fully grown plant. For example, scientists estimate broccoli sprouts contain at least ten times the antioxidant power of mature broccoli. During sprouting, the activity of enzymes increases dramatically, converting the starch into simple sugars, protein into amino acids and fats into fatty acids. These processes in effect pre-digest the seed, making it much easier for us to break down and absorb the nutrients. Whatever the content of the sprouts (and they will of course differ from one to the other), the key is freshness. If you let sprouts develop leaves and expose them to sunshine so they turn green, you'll have a fresh source of chlorophyll – the substance that makes plants green, which is renowned for its cleansing, anti-inflammatory and rejuvenating properties.

grow your own sprouts

GROWING MY OWN BEAN AND SEED SPROUTS REMINDS ME OF THE EXCITEMENT OF GROWING CRESS AS A SMALL CHILD — ON A BED OF COTTON WOOL IN A DARK CUPBOARD. IT'S REMARKABLY EASY AND A REWARDING WAY TO GROW SOME OF YOUR OWN FOOD — ESPECIALLY FOR ANYONE WHO IS A FRUSTRATED, GARDENLESS GARDENER. YOU CAN BUY SPECIALLY DESIGNED TRAYS AND JARS FOR GROWING SPROUTS FROM HEALTH FOOD SHOPS, BUT HERE'S A SIMPLE ALTERNATIVE.

about 2 tbsp **seeds***, such as mung beans, aduki, sunflower seeds, alfalfa, broccoli or radish per jar*

Punch several holes in the lid of a large, clean jar with a skewer. Put your chosen seeds into the jar. Use just one type per jar, as they grow at different rates. Soak the seeds in plenty of water overnight.

In the morning, drain the water out and rinse the seeds with fresh water, again draining out as much water as possible.

Put the jar in a dark cupboard. Each night and morning, rinse and drain the seeds again until they have sprouted and grown little roots.

After 3–6 days, depending on the type of seed and the warmth, the seeds will be ready to eat. Once they are ready you can store them in the fridge for up to 4 days, but throw them out if they start to turn brown any sooner.

Use in salads or just as a snack. If they have developed little leaves, as broccoli and alfalfa will, leave them on a windowsill for half a day to turn the leaves green before you put them in the fridge.

wonderfoods green salad

WITH SO MANY WONDERFUL INGREDIENTS AVAILABLE, THERE'S NO EXCUSE FOR
SERVING A MUNDANE GREEN SALAD BASED ON THE UBIQUITOUS ICEBERG LETTUCE.
THE TASTES AND TEXTURES IN THIS SALAD ARE AMAZING.

2 handfuls of baby **spinach**
  leaves
handful of **dandelion** leaves
handful of **watercress**
1 thin slice of **cabbage**,
  shredded
handful of whatever
  sprouts you have
$^1/_3$ **cucumber**, sliced
3 spring **onions**, trimmed
  and sliced
1 **avocado**, peeled, stoned
  and chopped
1 tbsp **pumpkin seeds**
FOR THE DRESSING
1 tsp Dijon mustard
1 small **garlic** clove, peeled
  and crushed
1 tbsp cider vinegar or
  balsamic vinegar
3 tbsp olive oil
fine sea salt
freshly ground black pepper

Trim and wash the spinach, dandelion and
watercress leaves, pat dry and place in a large
bowl with the cabbage, sprouts, cucumber, spring
onions and avocado.

To make the dressing, shake the mustard,
garlic and vinegar together in a screw-topped jar.
Add the olive oil and a little salt and pepper and
shake again.

Dress the salad just before you eat it and
sprinkle with the pumpkin seeds. It goes
wonderfully with barbecued fish or meat.

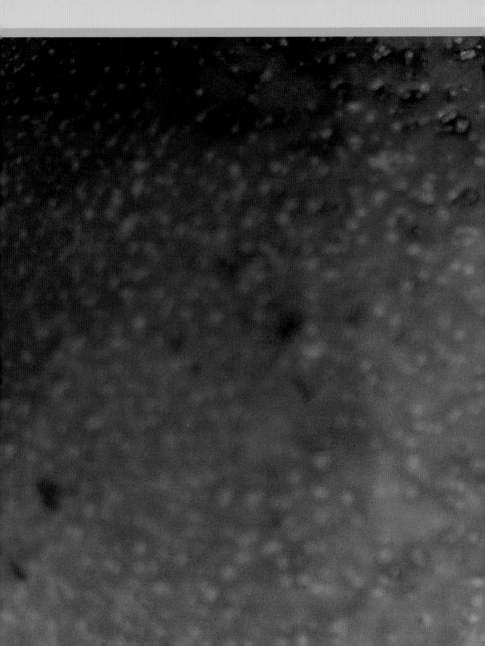

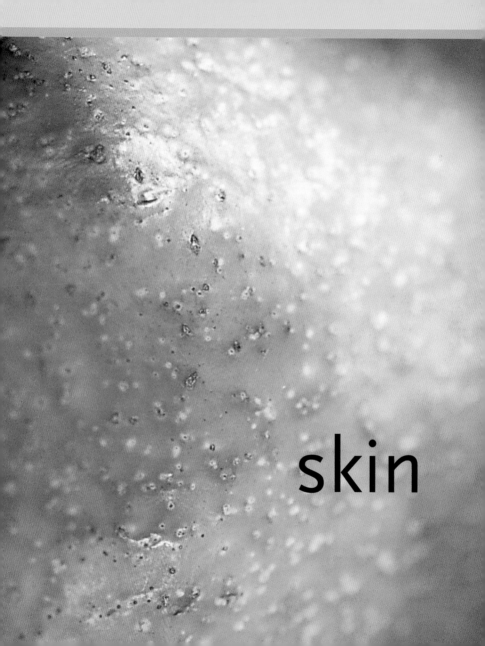

skin

We spend a lot of time and money nourishing, beautifying and treating our skin from the outside – with moisturisers and all those creams that promise to reduce the signs of ageing. But your skin's best chances may lie in your kitchen. You can slap on all the moisturiser you like, but if you are not feeding your skin the right nutrients it's going to remain a Sisyphean task!

Dry skin is a common complaint, but just by eating the wonderfoods in this chapter and throughout the book that contain healthy fats, you can go a long way to 'oiling' your skin from the inside out. Fats in nuts, seeds, avocados and fish can be incorporated into the cell membranes to keep them 'moisturised'. The second advantage to that is that the cells hold on to water better, leaving them nicely plump. One of the most important things to consume for good skin is water – not a wonderfood as such, but of course, essential to life. Think grapes rather than raisins – and that's what you want on the surface of your body, not to mention your internal 'skins' such as those in your gut and lungs.

Healthy skin is also dependent on a good supply of nutrients for the new skin cells to multiply in the deep layers and push through to the surface appropriately. Without enough zinc or vitamin A, for example, this won't take place properly, let alone when you need a wound to heal. Vitamins C and E are also fundamental for the structure of healthy skin.

Many skin problems like rashes, eczema and psoriasis involve inflammation, so nutrients that help counter this, such as healthy fats and vitamins, can help to relieve some of the symptoms. Another contributory factor to certain skin conditions – acne and psoriasis, for example – are congested bowels, so keeping them moving is important.

External factors, not least sun exposure, can also have a significant impact on the health of your skin. We do need our skin to see some sunlight for good health in order for the body to produce vitamin D, for example. However, excessive tanning under harsh sunlight or by artificial means is known to age the skin and even contribute to skin cancer. Also, the condition of your skin is affected by the substances it comes into contact with – cleaning products around the house, for example – as well as the actual skin care products you use. These can trigger allergic reactions or dry out skin. So watch what you do to your skin externally and eat skin-enhancing wonderfoods that nourish you from the inside to give you glowing skin.

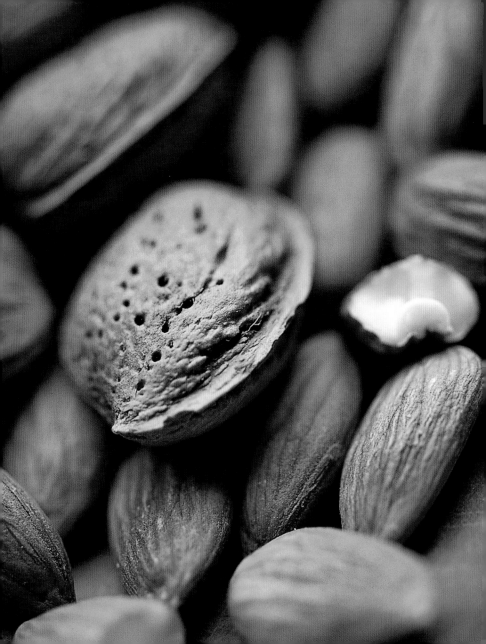

almonds

Nuts are in effect a seed – a concentrated package of goodness waiting to feed a newborn plant as it sprouts – and almonds happen to be one of the best. They are a good source of protein, especially for vegetarians, as well as fibre, B vitamins, vitamin E, calcium, magnesium, iron and zinc. Almonds have long been used in beauty care, and quite rightly. They are the nut with the highest fibre, which contributes to better elimination of waste products from the body, helping to keep the skin clear. Their vitamin E content plays an important role in skin, inside and out – helping to keep it elastic and to repair it if it is damaged. Almonds also contain monounsaturated fats and plant sterols, both of which help reduce the risk of heart disease. The magnesium in almonds is a useful muscle relaxant and needed to make energy. However, anyone who is susceptible to cold sores or other herpes infections should avoid almonds as they are rich in the amino acid arginine, which promotes the activation of the virus.

orange almond torte

THIS RICH CAKE IS HEAVENLY — AND YOU CAN FORGIVE YOURSELF ALL THE SUGAR
AND EGGS BECAUSE YOU ONLY NEED A THIN SLICE TO FEEL SATISFIED.

2 large **oranges**
170g caster sugar
200g ground **almonds**
4 **eggs**
juice of ½ **lemon**
½ tsp baking powder

Put the whole, unpeeled oranges in a pan and add cold water to cover. Bring to the boil, cover and simmer for 2 hours. Drain the oranges and leave them to cool.

Preheat the oven to 180°C/Gas 4. Grease a 23cm round cake tin and line with non-stick baking parchment. Cut the oranges into chunks and remove the pips, then tip them into a blender or food processor. Add the remaining ingredients and process until evenly blended, then pour the mixture into the cake tin. Bake for 45–60 minutes until risen and firm.

Turn the torte out on to a wire rack to cool. It's delicious served warm as a dessert with yoghurt or soured cream, but equally good eaten cold.

baked stuffed peaches

YOU CAN DO AN ALCOHOL-FREE VERSION OF THIS FOR CHILDREN OR
TEETOTALLERS, USING APPLE JUICE INSTEAD OF THE BRANDY.

1 heaped tbsp ground
  almonds
2 amaretti biscuits, crushed
2 tbsp brandy
4 ripe peaches, halved and
  stoned
*16 **almonds***
*100–150ml **apple** juice*

Preheat the oven to 180°C/Gas 4. In a bowl, mix together the ground almonds, crushed biscuits and brandy.

Put the peach halves, skin-side down, on a baking tray. Put a spoonful of the almond mixture into each cavity and top with two almonds. Pour enough apple juice into the dish to cover the bottom and bake for 30 minutes.

Serve the peaches warm, with natural yoghurt, vanilla ice cream or cream.

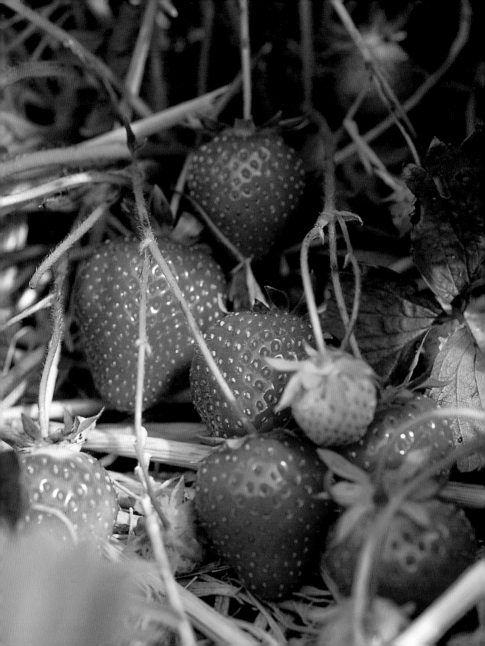

SKIN

strawberries

It is no coincidence that the Latin name for the world's most popular berry is *fragaria*, referring to its fragrance. And it's not only the taste that is fantastic. Just by eating five strawberries you could get your recommended daily intake of vitamin C, which is not only needed to protect against colds and cancer but also for clear skin and skin healing. Strawberries are similarly rich in the lesser-known vitamin K, needed for healthy bones and blood clotting. Their intense colour is due to anthocyanin, which protects all the body's cells, including skin, from oxidant damage that contributes to chronic diseases such as heart disease and cancer. Anthocyanins help curb inflammation in conditions like eczema, asthma and arthritis, too. Another antioxidant with anti-cancer properties in strawberries (and most other berries) is ellagic acid. The body's own antioxidant enzyme, superoxide dismutase, relies on manganese and this is also found in strawberries. The fruit's antioxidants have also been shown to help protect the brain from age-related decline.

artichoke & strawberry salad

I ALWAYS FEEL THERE'S SOMETHING LUXURIOUS ABOUT THIS SALAD THAT BELIES ITS SIMPLICITY. ADJUST THE DRESSING INGREDIENTS TO YOUR TASTE, ADDING A LITTLE MORE ORANGE JUICE, FOR EXAMPLE, IF YOU WANT A MORE TANGY FLAVOUR.

large handful of baby
  spinach, washed
large handful of rocket
  leaves, washed
4 **artichoke** hearts, cut into
  pieces
12 **walnuts**
8 **strawberries**, sliced
FOR THE DRESSING
8 medium-large ripe
  strawberries
1 tbsp **walnut** oil
juice of ¹/₂ **orange**
freshly ground black pepper

To make the dressing, whiz all the ingredients together in a blender until smooth.

Just before serving, combine the spinach and rocket leaves in a salad bowl. Add the artichoke hearts, walnuts and sliced strawberries, pour over the strawberry dressing and toss lightly.

appreciating strawberries

I DERIVE A SPECIAL PLEASURE FROM PICKING AND EATING A FRESH STRAWBERRY OFF THE PLANT IN THE GARDEN, ESPECIALLY IF IT'S OF THE SMALL, WILD VARIETY. OR POPPING A FRESH, ORGANIC ONE STRAIGHT INTO MY MOUTH FROM THE PUNNET. FOR ME, EVEN CREAM RUINS THE EXPERIENCE, SO THERE'S USUALLY NOT MUCH I WANT TO DO TO A FRESH STRAWBERRY.

That said, here are a few simple ways of enjoying them:

- Blend with banana, or pretty much any fruit to make a smoothie for breakfast or a snack.
- Slice and layer with blueberries and natural yoghurt.
- Chop and toss with orange juice, cinnamon and a drop of maple syrup, then roll in a buckwheat pancake.
- Blend a few strawberries with a little balsamic vinegar and a splash of olive oil to make a salad dressing.

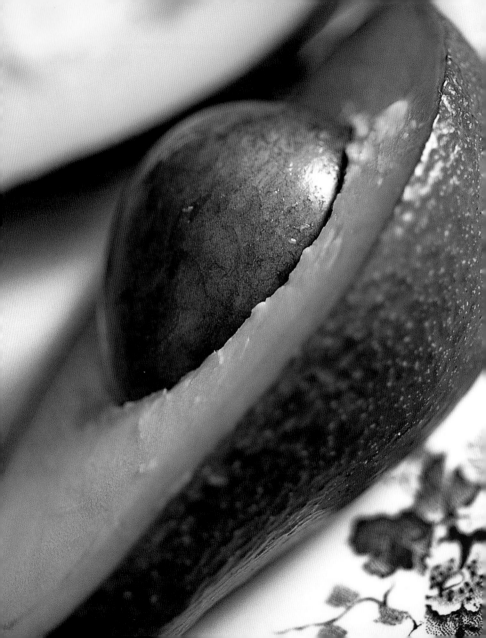

avocado

A member of the laurel family, the avocado tree produces pretty much the most nutritious fruit in the world. The name is derived from the Aztec word for testicle tree, apparently not owing to the shape of the fruit but because avocados have a reputation for exciting passion! They are loaded with heart healthy monounsaturated fat, fibre, vitamin E, folic acid, iron, vitamin B3 and potassium. Vitamin E is needed to keep the skin soft and supple. As if this was not enough, avocados are also the number one fruit source of beta-sitosterol, a substance that protects against cancer and can reduce total cholesterol. They also surpass other fruits in the antioxidant lutein, which studies have shown helps to protect people from cataracts, cardiovascular disease and prostate cancer. Avocados are easily digested, and their high fat content means that they are broken down slowly, which is useful for diabetics. They are also one of the richest sources of potassium, which is essential for healthy blood pressure, muscle contraction and nerve messaging.

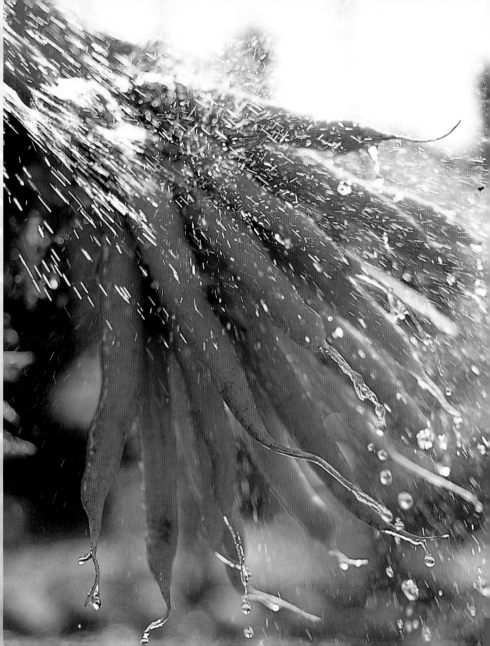

carrot

Ye old faithful carrot – common, inexpensive, versatile, vivid orange and renowned for helping you see in the dark; although apparently original carrots from central Asia were purple and not so sweet. Carrots' reputation for helping eye sight is down to their astoundingly high levels of beta carotene, which the body can convert to vitamin A for use in the skin, gut and immune system, as well as the eyes. Vitamin A, once in the retina of the eye, is turned into rhodopsin, a purple pigment that's needed for night vision. On top of that, beta carotene's antioxidant powers help protect against macular degeneration and cataracts. Beta carotene is just one carotenoid in carrots; another is alpha carotene which, with its beta cousin, helps reduce the risk of cancer and heart disease. Carrots are easy to digest, especially when cooked, and loaded with fibre, which is soothing for the digestive tract and boosts detoxification. Another boost for the skin comes from the mineral silica, as well as the vitamin C in carrots.

carrot salad

THIS MAKES AN INTERESTING SIDE SALAD, OR A GREAT LUNCH EATEN SIMPLY WITH
A CAN OF TUNA.

*3 medium **carrots**, peeled
and grated
small handful of shredded
cabbage
3 spring **onions**, trimmed
and finely sliced
1 tbsp roughly chopped
parsley
small handful of dried
seaweed, rehydrated
1–2 tbsp olive oil
juice of 1/2 **lemon**
1 tbsp toasted **sunflower
seeds***

Toss all the ingredients together in a large bowl
just before you eat.

carrot & ginger soup

THERE ARE SO MANY VARIATIONS ON THE CARROT SOUP THEME — THIS IS ONE FOR
THOSE WHO LIKE THE HOT TASTE OF GINGER, WHICH CUTS THROUGH THE
SWEETNESS OF THE CARROT PERFECTLY.

1 tsp olive oil
1 medium **onion**, peeled
and chopped
2 **garlic** cloves, peeled and
crushed
1 level tsp mustard powder
2.5cm piece fresh root
ginger, peeled and
grated
freshly ground black pepper
pinch of salt
1 litre vegetable or chicken
stock
6 medium-large **carrots**,
peeled and chopped
2 **celery** sticks, finely sliced
2 tbsp roughly chopped
parsley
natural **yoghurt**, to serve

Heat the olive oil in a large saucepan and soften
the onion and garlic with the mustard powder,
ginger, pepper and salt, adding 2 or 3 tbsp stock
after a minute or so. After another 2–3 minutes,
add the carrots and celery, stirring well. Pour in
the rest of the stock, bring to the boil, then cover
and leave to simmer for about 40 minutes.

When it is ready, whiz the soup until smooth in
a blender, or using a hand-held stick blender in the
pan. Stir in the chopped parsley, saving a little for
garnish and reheat the soup gently if you need to.

Pour into soup bowls and swirl a spoonful of
yoghurt through each portion. Sprinkle with the
reserved chopped parsley and serve.

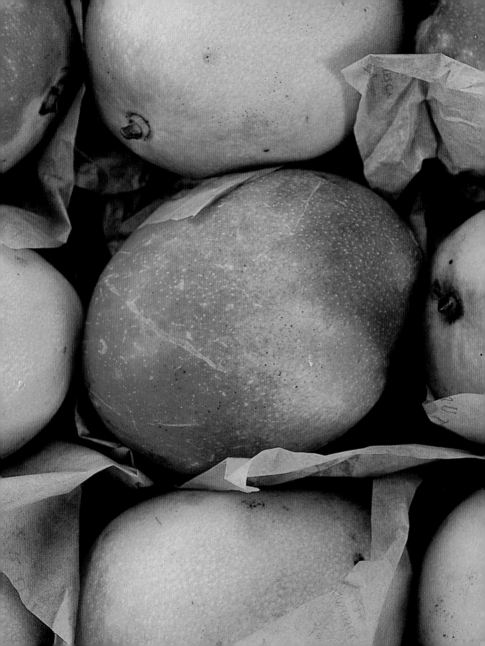

mango

Described by an Indian poet as 'sealed jars of honey', mangoes have been cultivated in India for 4,000 years or more. The fragrant, sweet flesh of a juicy mango has to be one of the most sensational taste experiences. And, unlike most sweet delights, mangoes are wonderfully good for you. Their bright orange-yellow colour gives away their beta carotene content. This is the plant form of vitamin A, which is needed for clear, unblemished skin, healthy lungs and intestines, and overall immunity. It complements the vitamin C in the fruit, which is important for the body to produce collagen, a protein in our skin and all connective tissue. Mangoes are a rich source of other antioxidants such as quercetin, which helps protect against allergies and respiratory problems. Like papaya, they contain enzymes that assist the digestion of food and cleansing of the bowel. They are also a good source of iron, potassium and magnesium, not to mention tryptophan, which the body can convert to the mood hormone, serotonin.

mango & pineapple salsa

I LIKE THIS TANGY, REFRESHING SALSA WITH PLAINLY GRILLED FISH, BUT IT'S ALSO
A GREAT WAY TO SPICE UP A TENDER, POACHED CHICKEN BREAST.

2 ripe but firm **mangoes**
1/2 ripe **pineapple**, peeled,
    cored and chopped
1/2 red **onion**, peeled and
    finely sliced
1cm piece fresh root **ginger**,
    peeled and grated
1 **garlic** clove, peeled and
    crushed
1 small red chilli, finely
    sliced
handful of coriander (leaves
    and stalks), roughly
    chopped
juice of 3 **limes**
2 tsp **sesame** oil

Peel and chop the mangoes over a salad bowl to
catch any runaway juice, tipping the fruit into the
bowl and discarding the stone. Add the pineapple,
onion, ginger, garlic, chilli and coriander and toss
together. Drizzle with the lime juice and sesame
oil, toss to mix and serve piled on top of grilled
fish or chicken.

mango in the buff

AS A CHILD, WHENEVER WE HAD THE LUXURY OF A MANGO, NOT A BIT WAS
WASTED. WE STRIPPED DOWN TO OUR UNDIES, SO AS NOT TO GET IN A MESS, AND
ATE THEM AT A TABLE, FROM WHICH WE COULD EVEN LICK THE JUICE AFTERWARDS!
YOU MAY NOT STRIP TO EAT YOUR MANGOES (NEITHER DO I THESE DAYS) BUT
THEY ARE SO SCENTED AND PRECIOUS, IT'S A SHAME TO ADULTERATE THEM MUCH.
FOR THIS 'RECIPE', ALL YOU NEED IS A MANGO AND YOUR TASTE BUDS ON ALERT.

1 *mango*

Firmly squeeze the mango in your hands,
massaging the flesh inside its skin until it feels
soft and separated from the stone. Only then, bite
a small, pea-sized hole in the top and noisily suck
out the molten flesh, squeezing it upwards to the
hole. When you really can't get another drop out,
tear back the skin and scrape your teeth along the
inside of each piece. Lastly scrape the stone until
your teeth are filled with shreds of mango hair and
the stone is dry!

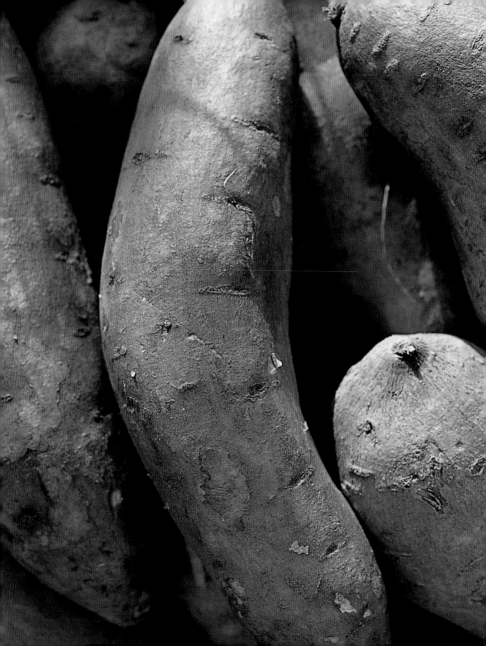

sweet potato

Unrelated to the common potato, the sweet potato is part of the morning glory family and grows on a vine. It is also much more nutritious. There are over 400 varieties but the orange-fleshed, pink-skinned sweet potatoes – also known by their Maori name *kumara* – are a great source of antioxidants. The more orange, the more abundant is the beta carotene, the plant form of vitamin A. As such they are beneficial for the skin, eyes and lungs, and along with the vitamin C in the vegetable, they provide support for the immune system. The sweetness comes from easily digestible sugars that make them a good source of energy, the release of which is somewhat tempered by the fibre content. The easy digestibility means that sweet potatoes are good for any inflammation in the gut, including ulcers. Ideally, cook them in their skins to maximise the conservation of nutrients. Sweet potatoes are wonderfully versatile and can be boiled, baked, roasted, steamed, mashed, and used in both savoury and sweet dishes.

sweet potato rösti

THESE RÖSTI ARE GREAT WITH GRILLED, SPICED FISH, SUCH AS TUNA OR SARDINES
AND A WONDERFOODS GREEN SALAD (PAGE 111). ALTERNATIVELY YOU CAN CRUMBLE
SOME GOAT'S CHEESE INTO AND ON TOP OF THEM AND MAKE SMALLER PATTIES TO
SERVE AS A STARTER...OR MAKE LARGER ONES FOR A VEGGIE MAIN COURSE.

2 medium **sweet potatoes**,
    scrubbed
1 medium **onion**, peeled
    and grated
1cm piece fresh root **ginger**,
    peeled and grated
1 **egg**, beaten
fine sea salt
freshly ground black pepper
a little olive oil

Preheat the oven to 200°C/Gas 6. Coarsely grate
the potatoes and then squeeze out as much
moisture as you can, using a tea towel. Tip the
grated potatoes into a bowl and mix with the
onion, ginger, egg, salt and pepper.

Oil a baking tray with olive oil. Form the potato
mix into four even patties, about 1cm thick, and
put them on the oiled tray. Carefully turn the
patties over (so the tops and bottoms are both
lightly oiled) and bake them for 25 minutes until
golden brown and crisp.

balsamic baked sweet potatoes

COOKED LIKE THIS, SWEET POTATOES MAKE A GREAT SIDE DISH TO ANY ROAST
MEAT, CHICKEN OR FISH. OR THEY CAN BE EATEN AS A MAIN MEAL WITH A
TOPPING SUCH AS AVOCADO CREAM (PAGE 127).

*4 small-medium **sweet
potatoes**, scrubbed
2 tbsp balsamic vinegar
4–6 **thyme** sprigs
freshly ground black pepper*

Preheat the oven to 180°C/Gas 4 (or a slightly
higher temperature is ok if you're using the oven
to roast meat). Toss the sweet potatoes in a
roasting dish with 1 tbsp balsamic vinegar and half
the thyme sprigs; season with pepper. Bake until
they feel soft all the way through when tested with
a skewer, about 40 minutes depending on size.

Slit the potatoes lengthways, cutting them
halfway through. Drizzle a little balsamic vinegar
into the opening and add a few thyme leaves.

sex

You may want to stop reading now, as I have possibly got you to this chapter under a false impression. The wonderfoods herein will not, I'm afraid, acquire you a good sex life or even sex at all (although a nice box of chocolates works for some people, hence its inclusion). There are, however, ingredients here that are known to help fertility and/or hormonal balance in the body.

For many reasons, mainly environmental, dietary and stress-related, more and more people are finding it difficult to conceive. Obviously, if you are having trouble, working with a professional is a sensible step. Before you get to that stage though, maximising not only your fertility but also your chances of conceiving a healthy baby can be done at least in part by optimising your nutrient intake. Low levels of zinc and vitamin E, for example (both found in seeds), have been linked to infertility. What's more, having good levels of essential nutrients means your body is less likely to hold on to harmful substances like lead, which can interfere with the hormonal system, amongst others.

Many women who suffer from premenstrual symptoms will give testament to the importance of dietary measures in helping to reduce their monthly pain, cravings and mood swings. Eating a range of wonderfoods (including small amounts of dark chocolate!) and avoiding caffeine and sugar make a significant difference in relieving such symptoms. Menopausal women also regularly find debilitating symptoms such as hot flushes, night sweats, fatigue and low moods can be lessened by the careful use of dietary strategies and herbal remedies (best taken under the guidance of a qualified herbalist). Men can benefit from these wonderfoods, too. Increasingly common disorders of the prostate gland have been shown to respond positively to certain nutrients, such as those in pumpkin seeds and tomatoes.

And on a more serious note about sex itself, if you really do find your libido is down, living on a diet of wonderfoods in general, steering clear of foods and drinks that 'stress' the body (sugar, caffeine, alcohol, junk food), handling stresses in your life, getting enough sleep and dealing with any underlying emotional issues – especially with your partner, of course – can go a long way to making you feel horny.

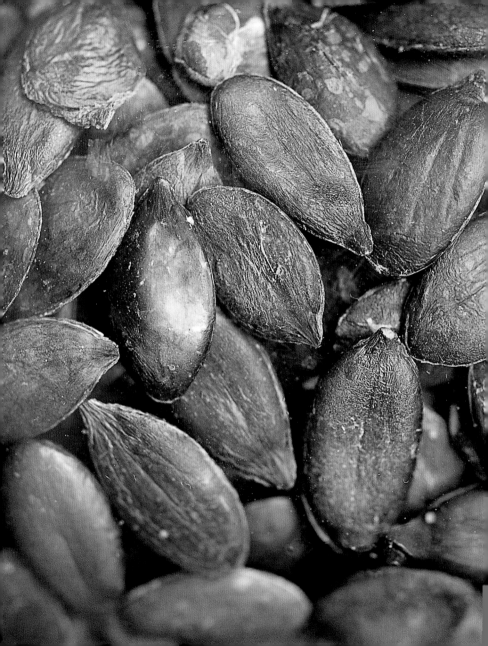

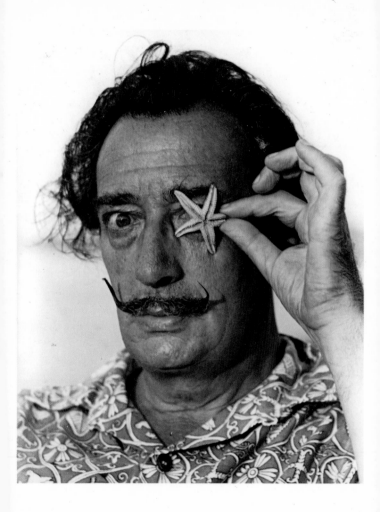

both 2017

Wishing you

a very Happy

— and Heathy!

Produït per Das Edicions SA

d.a.s.
edicions

New Year —

love from Mum &

Dad.

I love this book!
(try the carrot soup :-)

Salvador Dalí, 1958
Foto: Xavier Miserachs

pumpkin seeds

Creamy and nutty, the seeds scooped from your Halloween pumpkin are about the most nutritious and delicious you can buy. They're not only rich in essential fatty acids (EFAs) but also full of important micronutrients, like vitamin E, iron and magnesium – all needed for good sexual health and fertility. EFAs are important in maintaining smooth soft, elastic skin that holds water well, so it doesn't become easily dehydrated. The incorporation of EFAs into cell membranes means they are better able to receive hormonal messages. Pumpkin seeds are particularly rich in zinc, a mineral needed for sexual function, defence against infections, proper growth and the development of new cells. Zinc and EFAs have been linked to helping reduce prostate enlargement. The calcium and magnesium in pumpkin seeds are needed for healthy bones, nerves and muscles, while the cucurbitacins they contain have anti-inflammatory and anti-cancer properties. Pumpkin seeds are a good source of protein for vegetarians and contain vitamin B6, which has countless roles, including helping hormone balance in women.

green light salad

THIS IS A STAPLE GREEN SALAD IN OUR HOUSEHOLD, WITH OTHER GREENS FROM
THE GARDEN ADDED IN SUMMER, SUCH AS ROCKET, SORREL AND LOVAGE. YOU CAN
EVEN THROW IN SOME HAZELNUTS OR CHICKPEAS TO MAKE IT A SUBSTANTIAL
LUNCH IN ITS OWN RIGHT.

2 handfuls of baby **spinach**,
    washed
2 handfuls of **watercress**,
    trimmed and washed
10–12 **basil** leaves
2 spring **onions**, trimmed
    and finely sliced
1 tbsp **pumpkin seeds**
1 **avocado**, peeled, stoned
    and chopped
1 tbsp olive oil
juice of ½ **lemon**

Toss all the ingredients together in a large bowl
and eat immediately. Or assemble the leaves,
spring onions and pumpkin seeds in advance,
adding the avocado, olive oil and lemon juice at
the last minute.

seed-crusted monkfish in parma ham

BECAUSE OF THE LIGHT, MEATINESS OF MONKFISH, IT CAN EASILY CARRY THE
FLAVOURS OF OILY PUMPKIN SEEDS AND SALTY HAM.

4 tbsp **pumpkin seeds**
2 **shallots**, *peeled and quartered*
12 **basil** *leaves (or more)*
juice of 1 **lemon**
4 *pieces of* **monkfish** *fillet, each about 150g*
4 *slices of Parma ham*

Preheat the oven to 180°C/Gas 4. Using a pestle and mortar, grind the pumpkin seeds with the shallots, basil and lemon juice to a rough paste.

Wrap each piece of monkfish in a slice of Parma ham and lay in a baking dish. Smear the tops with the seed paste. Pour a little water into the dish, just enough to thinly cover the bottom. Bake for 15–20 minutes until the fish is cooked through. Serve with a salad or steamed green veg.

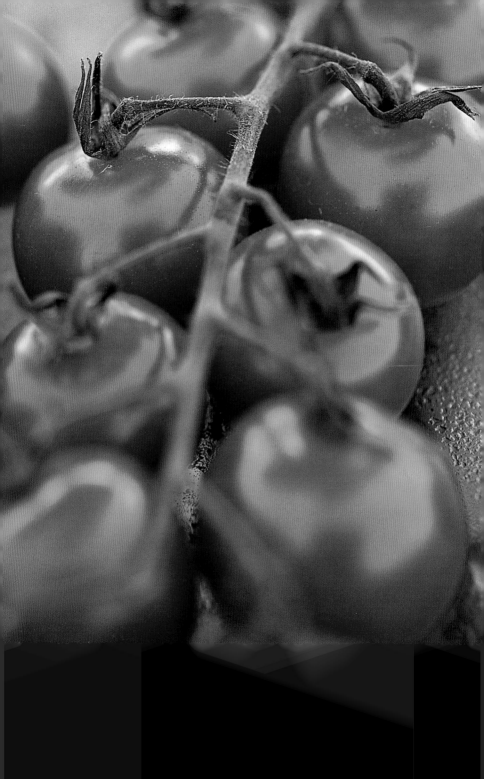

tomato

Originally from the lowlands between the Andes and the Pacific Ocean, the tomato is one of the most commonly eaten wonderfoods. Unlike many fruits and vegetables, some of the benefits of tomatoes are increased when they are cooked. This is because the heating process helps release certain nutrients, notably lycopene, phytoene and phytofluene – carotenoids that give tomatoes their red colour and protective powers. Lycopene has been shown to protect against cancer (especially prostate) and guard the skin and eyes from sun damage. As these carotenoids are fat soluble, they need to be eaten with a little fat to be absorbed (tomatoes with olive oil, for example). The rich vitamin C and potassium content of tomatoes makes them helpful in combating cardiovascular disease. But this fruit has not always been recognised as beneficial to health. Several 16th–19th century herbal treatises pronounced the tomato 'injurious' and 'unwholesome', possibly because like peppers and aubergines, tomatoes contain solanine, which in some people exacerbates the symptoms of arthritis.

frittata tricolore

NAMED AFTER THE ITALIAN FLAG, THIS FRITTATA CAN BE EATEN HOT AS SOON AS IT'S COOKED, OR COLD. YOU'LL NEED A FRYING PAN THAT IS SUITABLE TO USE BRIEFLY UNDER THE GRILL.

6 **eggs**
freshly ground black pepper
splash of olive oil
handful of **spinach**, washed
    and roughly chopped
2 medium **tomatoes**, sliced
4–6 **basil** leaves, torn
150g goat's cheese, sliced

Preheat the grill. Beat the eggs in a bowl with some pepper.

Heat the olive oil in a large frying pan over a medium heat, then pour in the beaten eggs. Scatter the spinach, tomatoes, basil and goat's cheese over the egg. Cook on the hob for about 3 minutes without stirring, then put it under a hot grill for a minute or so until the top is golden brown. Serve with a Sunny salad (page 218).

warm chickpea & tomato salad

THIS MAKES A GREAT MAIN COURSE IN ITSELF, OR YOU CAN SERVE IT WITH A
MIDDLE EASTERN DISH, SUCH AS CARROT FELAFEL (PAGE 183), AND A
WONDERFOODS GREEN SALAD (PAGE 111).

1 tbsp olive oil, plus extra
    to drizzle
1 red **onion**, peeled and
    finely sliced
3 **garlic** cloves, peeled and
    sliced
2 tsp freshly grated root
    ginger
1 tsp ground cumin
freshly ground black pepper
generous pinch of sea salt
2 x 400g cans **chickpeas**,
    drained
4–5 tbsp water
500g cherry **tomatoes**
100g baby **spinach** leaves,
    washed
natural **yoghurt**, to serve

Heat the olive oil in a large pan and toss in the
onion, garlic, ginger, cumin, pepper and salt.
Sauté for about 5 minutes, then add the chickpeas
and water. Stir well until most of the liquid has
evaporated, then add the tomatoes and leave to
cook for 3–4 minutes. Throw in the spinach leaves
and cook briefly until wilted.

Drizzle with a little more olive oil and serve
with natural yoghurt to dollop on top. Accompany
with wholemeal pitta or brown rice.

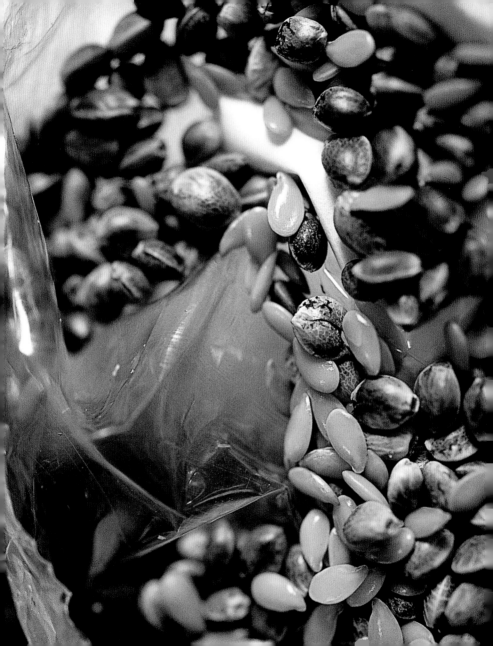

hemp seeds & linseed

If you think these seeds are simply bird food, think again. Both hemp seeds and linseed are loaded with omega 6 and omega 3 essential fatty acids (EFAs). These are needed for brain and nerve cells, and therefore important for pretty much all of our body functions, including memory and good moods. Hemp seeds are one of the richest plant sources of omega 3 fatty acids, which help keep blood from clotting excessively, and because of their anti-inflammatory properties, they are natural painkillers – useful for conditions like arthritis. Hemp seeds are also one of the only food sources of GLA, an omega 6 derivative prized for staving off PMS. Linseed (also known as flax) contain lignans, which have been linked to a lower risk of breast and prostate cancers. Like other seeds, hemp and linseed contain zinc, calcium and magnesium. To benefit from their nutrients, it's best to grind them in a coffee grinder otherwise they're not digested. Or to relieve constipation, soak a tablespoonful of linseed in a glass of water for a few hours and then drink the lot.

high five mix

THIS BLEND OF SEEDS, ONCE GROUND UP, CAN BE USED TO PUT A HEALTHY, NUTTY
TOPPING ON YOGHURT, CEREAL, SOUPS AND CASSEROLES. YOU WILL NEED TO KEEP
THE SEEDS IN SEALED JARS IN THE FRIDGE AS THE ESSENTIAL FATTY ACIDS (EFAs)
THEY CONTAIN ARE EASILY 'DAMAGED' OR OXIDISED BY HEAT AND LIGHT.

equal quantities of:
linseed *(flax seeds)*
pumpkin seeds
sunflower seeds
sesame seeds
hemp seeds

Grind a batch of mixed seeds in a coffee grinder –
kept solely for the purpose of course! You can do
this in advance if you like, provided you keep the
ground mix in an airtight jar in the fridge. Once
crushed, the seeds are even more susceptible to
turning rancid, so use within 2–3 weeks.

Scatter the seed mix over yogurt, cereal, soups
or casseroles – to add creaminess and goodness.

toasty seed snack

THIS IS A GREAT SNACK THAT CHILDREN WILL LOVE TOO. YOU CAN ALSO SCATTER IT OVER SALADS TO ADD CRUNCH. MAKE UP A BIG BATCH IN ADVANCE AND STORE IT IN AN AIRTIGHT CONTAINER.

*3 tbsp **pumpkin seeds***
*3 tbsp **sunflower seeds***
*2 tbsp **sesame seeds***
*2 tbsp **linseed** (flax seeds)*
1 tbsp tamari or soy sauce

Preheat the oven to 170°C/Gas 3¹/₂. Line a baking tray with baking parchment.

In a bowl, toss all the seeds together with the tamari so they are well coated. Scatter the seeds on the lined baking tray. Toast in the oven for 15 minutes, shaking the tray or stirring the seeds well a couple of times during cooking.

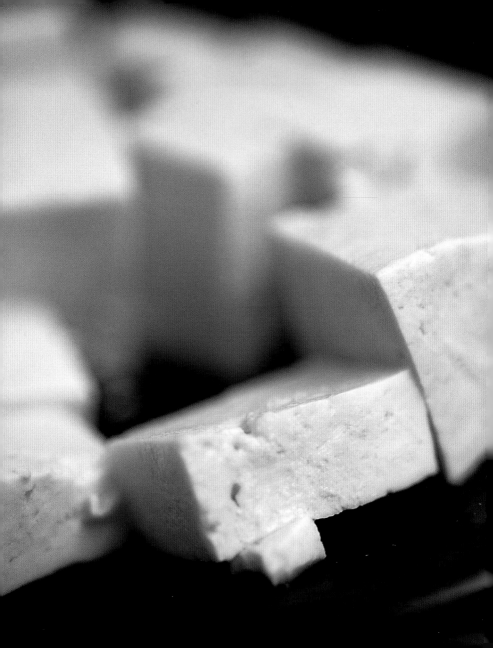

soya

Even if you're not vegetarian, you may well have soya in your diet in some form – perhaps tofu, soya milk, miso or tempeh. Soya milk is invaluable for those with a sensitivity to cow's milk; some babies are fed on soy-based formulas. For vegans and vegetarians, soya is a good source of first class protein – containing all the essential amino acids. It is also one of the richest natural sources of isoflavones, a type of phyto (plant) oestrogens. These are believed to help block the effect of hormone-disrupting chemicals in our environment, thought to cause problems such as premenstrual syndrome, polycystic ovaries, breast and prostate cancers. Phyto-oestrogens may also help if a woman is low in oestrogen, for example, at the menopause they can help to relieve symptoms. Other potential benefits are lowered cholesterol and a reduced risk of osteoporosis. Some studies suggest soya to be harmful, but two or three servings a week is fine, and probably good for you. Buy organic, to avoid genetically modified soya.

roast chicken noodle soup

THIS IS A WONDERFUL DISH TO MAKE WITH LEFTOVER CHICKEN OR DUCK. YOU
COULD USE RICE NOODLES INSTEAD OF SOBA IF YOU PREFER.

2 boneless **chicken** breasts
(with skin)
2 tsp Chinese five spice
powder
1 tbsp sweet chilli sauce
750ml water
3 tbsp miso (**soya** paste)
2.5cm piece fresh root
ginger or galangal,
sliced
2 red chillies, deseeded and
sliced
2 lemongrass stalks, sliced
150g dried soba
(**buckwheat**) noodles
2 spring **onions**, trimmed
and sliced
juice of 1 **lime**
2 handfuls of **mung sprouts**
(see page 110)
2 tbsp coriander leaves, torn

Preheat the oven to 180°C/Gas 4. Smear the
chicken breasts with the five spice powder and
sweet chilli sauce, place in a small roasting pan
and roast in the oven for 25 minutes or until they
are cooked through.

Meanwhile, bring the water to the boil in a
large pan and turn the heat down to a simmer.
Scoop out half a mugful and stir the miso paste
into this, then pour it back into the pan.

Crush the ginger, chillies and lemongrass
using a pestle and mortar, then add to the soup
(or you can just throw them in sliced). Simmer for
about 15 minutes, then add the soba noodles,
spring onions and lime juice. Cook for about 6–8
minutes until the noodles are just tender.

Meanwhile, slice the chicken into bite-sized
pieces. Ladle the soup into warm bowls and divide
the chicken and mung sprouts among them.
Scatter over the coriander to serve.

sesame soya stir-fry

I LIKE TO EAT THIS STIR-FRY ON A PILE OF RICE NOODLES THAT HAVE BEEN TOSSED WITH SESAME OIL AND FRESH CORIANDER LEAVES.

250g firm **tofu**, cubed
1 tbsp soy sauce
1cm piece fresh root **ginger**, peeled and finely sliced
1 **garlic** clove, peeled and finely sliced
1 tbsp sweet chilli sauce
splash of **sesame** oil
4 spring **onions**, trimmed and chopped
1 **red pepper**, cored, deseeded and cut into strips
1 **carrot**, peeled and cut into thin strips
handful of mangetout
2–3 tbsp water
1 tbsp finely chopped coriander leaves
2 tbsp **sesame seeds**

Put the tofu in a bowl with the soy sauce, ginger, garlic and chilli sauce. Toss to mix and set aside to marinate while you prepare the vegetables.

Heat a wok or large frying pan and add a splash of sesame oil. Add the tofu with its marinade and toss continuously over a high heat for a couple of minutes. Remove the tofu with a slotted spoon and set aside on a plate.

Add the spring onions, red pepper, carrot and mangetout to the wok, toss quickly and then add 2–3 tbsp water to 'steam-fry' the vegetables. Stir well over a high heat for about 2 minutes.

Add the chopped coriander and put the tofu back into the pan to reheat briefly, but don't let the vegetables become too soft. Sprinkle the stir-fry with sesame seeds to serve.

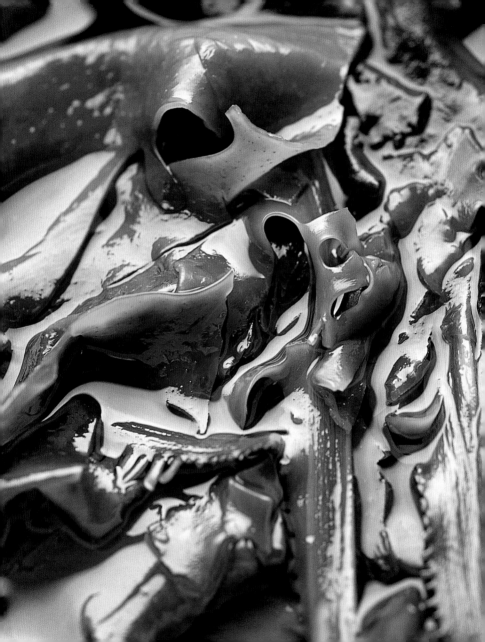

seaweed

It's the wafting weed that gives you the creeps as it brushes your leg in the sea, but seaweed is one of nature's true wonderfoods and it has been eaten for millennia – you will find it depicted in Egyptian hieroglyphs. Wild seaweed, or algae, is a great source of minerals and a powerful cleanser, as long as it hasn't been harvested from polluted waters. It's a very good source of iodine, which is an important player in the body's hormonal system. This mineral is needed to make the thyroid hormone that is responsible for dictating our body's metabolism, i.e. all its activities. An underactive thyroid is linked to fatigue and a low sex drive. The chlorophyll that makes seaweed green is a natural detoxifier and its alginic acid helps draw out waste. Seaweed also contains lignans, which have cancer-protective properties and it provides the full alphabet of essential minerals and vitamins – in a natural balance that enhances the synergy of the nutrients. We would all do well to include seaweed in our diet regularly.

crunchy summer salad

YOU CAN ADD SOME SHREDDED CABBAGE TO MAKE THIS SALAD EVEN CRUNCHIER.
SERVE IT AS A LIGHT STARTER, OR AS A SIDE DISH TO NOODLES OR A STIR-FRY.

small handful of dried
seaweed*, such as arame*
3 medium-large **carrots***,*
peeled and grated
3 spring **onions***, trimmed*
and finely sliced
about 10 coriander sprigs,
roughly chopped
2 tsp **sesame** *oil*
1 tbsp tamari or soy sauce
juice of 1–2 **limes***, to taste*
1 tbsp **sesame seeds**

Put the seaweed in a mug, pour on just about enough boiling water to cover and leave it to steep for 4–5 minutes. Meanwhile, in a large bowl, combine the carrots, spring onions and coriander.

When the seaweed is soft, drain it in a sieve, tossing to cool it off before adding to the salad. Add the sesame oil, tamari and lime juice (using more rather than less if you want a tangy flavour). Toss all the ingredients together well.

Just before serving, sprinkle the sesame seeds over the salad.

enjoying seaweed

IF YOU'RE NOT USED TO COOKING WITH SEAWEED, THE IDEA MAY INITIALLY SEEM A BIT DAUNTING, BUT IT IS REMARKABLY VERSATILE AND TASTY... NOT TO MENTION BEING A WONDERFOOD.

- Health food shops and some large supermarkets now sell a range of dried Japanese varieties, such as wakame, hijiki and arame. These need rehydrating before use and can be added to soups, stir-fries, stews or salads.
- You can also get dried European sea vegetables, like dulse or sea lettuce. Specialist greengrocers and fishmongers sometimes sell them non-dried, usually preserved in salt. Rinse these well and eat them raw in salads, stir-fries, omelettes or soups.
- Seaweed the windbreaker: when you're cooking beans or chickpeas, add a strip of kombu, a Japanese seaweed. It helps reduce the wind factor in the beans by making them more easily digestible.

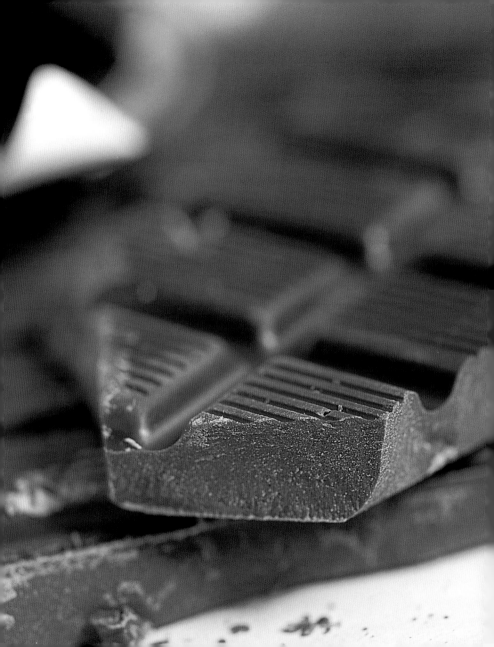

chocolate

It is said the Aztec emperor Montezuma drank chocolate daily to enhance his sexual prowess, though it would have been a very different drink from today. There's no clear reason why chocolate is considered sexy or romantic but the rich, sweetness blended with a light stimulant may be what makes it a lovers' favourite. Its divine properties are acknowledged in its classification: *Theobroma cacao* – theobroma meaning food of the gods. Chocolate's major ingredient, cocoa, is a source of theobromine, which mildly stimulates the nervous system. Chocolate contains small amounts of mood-enhancing phenethylamine, too. It also has a high content of antioxidants including polyphenolic flavonoids, which reduce inflammation, keep blood vessels healthy and lower the risk of cancer. That said, regular consumption of fats and sugars in chocolate is linked to health problems. So eat organic, dark chocolate, which contains more cocoa and therefore less sugar and fat. Chocolate is good for the soul and that makes it a wonderfood in my book!

baked banana choc split

THIS RECIPE CAN EVEN BE COOKED ON A BARBECUE – THE FIRST TIME I MADE IT
WAS UNDER A GLORIOUSLY STARRY NIGHT ON A BEACH IN SOUTH DEVON. IT
COULDN'T BE EASIER.

4 **bananas** (unpeeled)
12 squares of dark, organic
   chocolate
4 tbsp soured cream
16 **almonds**, roughly
   broken up

Preheat the oven to 180°C/Gas 4. Lay the bananas, still in their skins, on a baking tray and bake for 20–25 minutes until they are soft.

Lay each banana on its side on a plate and make a slit along most of the length through the skin and halfway through the banana. Squeeze the slit open by pushing up from the outside of the skin. Slip 3 pieces of chocolate into each slit and spoon on the soured cream.

Top with the almonds and serve immediately, as the chocolate melts.

chocolate fridge slice

CHILDREN WILL LOVE MAKING — AND EATING — THIS ONE. BIG CHILDREN TOO! YOU CAN USE ANY DRIED FRUIT YOU FANCY.

30g **almonds**, roughly broken up

30g **pumpkin seeds**

150g dried fruit, such as raisins, **apricots**, **papaya, berries**

50ml brandy (or orange juice)

180g dark, organic **chocolate**

50g unsalted butter

75g digestive biscuits, broken into small pieces

If you want to roast the almonds and pumpkin seeds to enhance their flavour, toss them in a dry frying pan for a few minutes until they brown a little and the pumpkin seeds pop. Leave to cool.

Cut larger dried fruits into small, raisin-sized pieces. Put all the fruit in a bowl, add the brandy, stir well and set aside to macerate.

Line a 20cm flan dish or cake tin with cling film, letting it overhang the rim. Melt the chocolate and butter together in a small pan over a very low heat — take care to avoid overheating.

Drain the dried fruit and tip into a bowl. Mix in the almonds, pumpkin seeds and biscuit pieces. Pour in the melted chocolate mix and stir it all together well. Pour the whole lot into the prepared dish and leave in the fridge overnight until firm. Serve in slices, as it is or with a little soured cream.

age

It won't come as any surprise that I'm not suggesting eating the foods in this section will turn back the clock for you, or enable your liver to cope with partying as you did when you were twenty! But there are legitimate, scientific reasons why these foods all fall under the age category of wonderfoods. They are all particularly high in naturally occurring chemicals with antioxidant properties.

Antioxidants counter the effect of oxidants, which are sometimes known as free radicals. Oxidants are highly reactive compounds that are produced when the body uses oxygen. The body has very sophisticated mechanisms in the form of antioxidant enzyme systems to go round mopping up after the oxidants. We are also exposed to oxidants in our environments, from car exhaust fumes, pesticides, sun radiation, smoking, alcohol, some medications, even burnt food.

Although oxidants are normal by-products of the body's workings and our surroundings, there is no doubt that excessive exposure is detrimental to health, particularly when coupled with insufficient exposure to antioxidants. In effect, oxidants multiply through a chain reaction, creating a cascade of damage, particularly to cell membranes and our cell reproductive blueprint, our DNA. Scientists have made clear links between oxidants and several degenerative diseases (such as heart disease, cancer, Alzheimer's) and the ageing process. Also linked to ageing is a decline in the body's immune system and a higher risk of infection; antioxidants can also help support immunity.

Common antioxidants are vitamins A, C and E, beta carotene, selenium, zinc and flavonoids. A good daily dose of these protective substances is crucial for good health and to minimise the ageing process. I'm not necessarily referring to ironing out those crow's feet or frown lines, but more the internal ageing of our bodies that leaves them not working quite as efficiently as they used to. And no amount of these foods is going to compensate for the set of genes you were born with, habits like smoking or other factors that contribute to ageing. The foods in this category need to be eaten alongside others throughout the book and even then, your diet is just one thing to consider in helping you age gracefully and in good health. Others are: getting sufficient sleep, exercising appropriately and not overeating. Whatever else you do, as long as you're eating good amounts of the foods in this section and other wonderfoods, at least you're maximising your chances of minimising ageing.

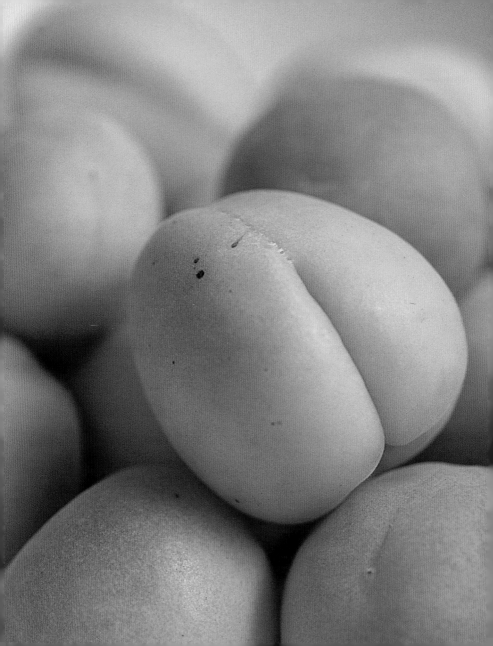

apricot

The softness of a ripe apricot may not yield the juiciest of flesh, but it certainly packs a punch with flavour and health. It is even said to have been the original nectar of the gods. Like other orange-coloured fruit and vegetables, apricots are a mine of beta carotene, which protects the skin and lungs from oxidation damage and supports a healthy immune system. Apricots are rich in fibre, so they can help relieve constipation and ward off digestive problems such as diverticulitis, particularly when eaten dried. Too much dried fruit, though, can cause bloating so stop yourself from eating too many – you probably wouldn't eat ten fresh apricots, so best not to eat ten dried ones in one go! Although fresh apricots are best eaten either alone, in smoothies, or desserts, the dried ones make an interesting addition to savoury meat or chicken dishes, as they are used in the Middle East. Most dried apricots are preserved with sulphur dioxide, so go for the darker, non-sulphured ones.

spiced apricots

THIS IS ONE OF THE MOST POPULAR, EASY AND HEALTHY DESSERTS I MAKE. IF YOU HAVE A PACKET OF DRIED APRICOTS IN THE CUPBOARD, YOU CAN RUSTLE IT UP AT SHORT NOTICE FOR GUESTS.

200g dried **apricots**
200ml water
100ml **apple** *juice*
3 star anise
10 **cardamom** *pods*

Put all the ingredients in a saucepan and bring to the boil. Cover and leave to simmer for at least an hour to get the most out of the spices, though less will do if you don't have the time. Take the lid off if you want to reduce the syrup further.

Serve with natural yoghurt or, if you're feeling more indulgent, vanilla ice cream.

apricot salsa

THIS FRESH, RAW 'CHUTNEY' GOES PERFECTLY WITH CHEESE AND ALL SORTS OF SAVOURY DISHES, SUCH AS CARROT FELAFEL (PAGE 183) AND PLAIN ROAST OR GRILLED CHICKEN AND MEAT. MAKE SURE THE APRICOTS ARE NICELY RIPE TO SWEETEN THE WHOLE MIX.

6 ripe **apricots**, stoned and finely chopped
1 tbsp capers, roughly chopped
2 **shallots** (or 1 small red **onion**), peeled and very finely diced
few **basil** leaves, roughly torn
juice of 1 **lemon** (or ½ if it's large)
pinch of ground **cinnamon**
2 tbsp olive oil
freshly ground black pepper

Mix all the ingredients together in a bowl. Ideally, leave for about an hour to allow the flavours to infuse, but the salsa still tastes fine if you serve it straight away.

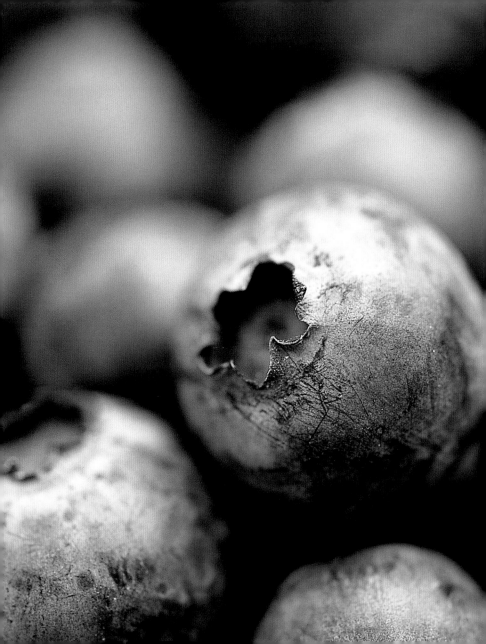

blueberries

Native Americans have known for centuries that juicy blueberries are remarkable. Sometimes called bilberries, they are an amazing source of antioxidants, particularly anthocyanidins, as are another dark relative, blackberries. These potent chemicals are protective in their own right against ageing caused by oxidant damage, but also help increase the potency of vitamin C. Studies have shown that blueberries can help to improve brain function and they have an affinity with the eyes, helping night vision and protecting against age-related macular degeneration, cataracts and glaucoma. Blueberries strengthen the entire vascular system (veins and arteries), making sure that all parts of the body get sufficient oxygen and vital nutrients. They also contain a substance called pterostilbene, which helps lower cholesterol and protect against cancer. The antioxidants in blueberries help protect our cellular support structure, collagen, from oxidant damage – so improving skin tone. Blueberries are also a good source of fibre.

blueberry cheesecake

YOU CAN VARY THIS CHEESECAKE BY USING ALL SORTS OF OTHER FRUIT, SUCH AS
RASPBERRIES, STRAWBERRIES OR STONED CHERRIES. IF YOU WANT A GLUTEN-FREE
DESSERT, OMIT THE BASE, MAKE $1\frac{1}{2}$ TIMES THE AMOUNT OF FILLING, SPOON INTO
A BOWL, TOP WITH THE BLUEBERRIES AND CHILL BEFORE SERVING.

FOR THE BASE
100g rolled **oats**
50g **almonds**, chopped
1 tbsp brown sugar or
    alternative equivalent
    (see page 10)
1 tsp ground **cinnamon**
80g butter, melted
FOR THE FILLING
300g cream cheese
2 tbsp amaretto liqueur
    (or water)
2 tbsp **lemon** juice
2 tbsp icing sugar
FOR THE TOPPING
300g **blueberries**

Preheat the oven to 180°C/Gas 4. For the base,
mix the oats, almonds, sugar and cinnamon
together on a large baking tray and toast in the
oven for 20–25 minutes. (I sometimes first grind
the oats in a blender for a minute – to make a
finer base.)

Meanwhile, prepare the topping. In a bowl,
whisk the cream cheese with the amaretto, lemon
juice and icing sugar until evenly blended.

When the base ingredients are toasted, stir in
the melted butter and press the mixture into the
bottom of a 23cm flan dish. Ideally leave it in the
fridge to set for a couple of hours.

Spread the cream cheese mixture over the base
and top with the blueberries. Refrigerate until
ready to serve.

mango incognito

YOU CAN BARELY MAKE OUT THE MANGO FROM THE COLOUR OF THIS DELICIOUS
SMOOTHIE, BUT THE TASTE CERTAINLY TELLS YOU IT'S THERE. THE GUAVA ADDS A
DIFFERENT DIMENSION ALTOGETHER, THOUGH YOU CAN USE APPLE IF YOU CAN'T
FIND GUAVA JUICE.

*3 handfuls of **blueberries***
*1 large **mango** (or 2 small ones)*
*5 tbsp natural **yoghurt***
*120ml guava juice (ideally, or **apple** juice)*

Whiz all the ingredients together in a blender and drink straight away, but not quickly!

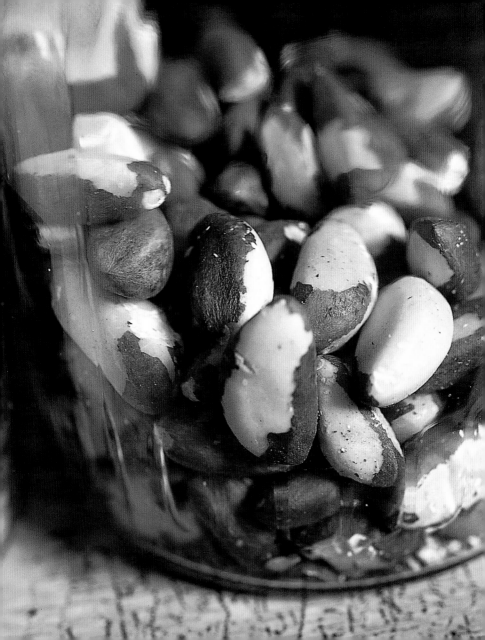

brazil nuts

Unlike much of the food we eat, Brazil nuts have yet to be grown successfully on plantations – they are harvested from huge, wild trees in the Latin American rainforest. The wedge shaped nuts form segments in fruits that are about the size of a large grapefruit. Brazil nuts are best known, nutritionally, for their rich selenium content. This mineral is needed to activate an enzyme in the body called glutathione peroxidase, which helps protect us against oxidants and the development of cancer cells. Studies have shown that a higher selenium intake is linked to a lower incidence of various types of cancer. Selenium is also needed by the immune system, for thyroid hormones to work properly and for healthy sperm. Brazil nuts are about 70% fat: half is oleic (as in olive oil) and much of the rest is omega 6 with some omega 3. Because of this, it is best to buy Brazils in their shells as the fat is prone to turn rancid and the nut keeps better in its natural case.

brazil nut & watercress pesto

THIS DELICIOUS SAUCE NOT ONLY GOES WITH PASTA, LIKE A REGULAR PESTO, BUT
ALSO WITH ANY GRILLED FISH OR MEAT.

16–20 **Brazil nuts**, shelled
2 **garlic** cloves, peeled
2 large handfuls of
  watercress, washed
150g Parmesan cheese,
  finely (and freshly)
  grated
juice of ½ **lemon**
freshly ground black pepper
3–4 tbsp olive oil (or more
  if needed)

Whiz the nuts, garlic, watercress, Parmesan,
lemon juice and a generous grinding of pepper
together in a blender, adding the olive oil a little at
a time until you have a smooth, fresh sauce.

Toss the pesto with freshly cooked pasta or
serve spooned over hot, grilled fish or meat.

carrot felafel

THESE ARE A LESS DENSE VERSION OF REAL, MIDDLE EASTERN CHICKPEA FALAFEL. THEY ARE GREAT SERVED WITH APRICOT SALSA (PAGE 175), NATURAL YOGHURT AND A WONDERFOODS GREEN SALAD (PAGE 111), OR ROLLED IN A WARM PITTA BREAD WITH A LITTLE TAHINI (SESAME PASTE), CHILLI SAUCE, TOMATOES AND CUCUMBER. FOR A VEGETARIAN MAIN COURSE, DOUBLE THE QUANTITIES LISTED.

125g **chickpeas** (cooked or canned, well drained)
1 small **onion**, peeled and quartered
1 **garlic** clove, peeled
handful of **parsley**
1/2 tsp ground cumin
1/2 tsp ground coriander
1/2 tsp cayenne pepper (or a dash of Tabasco sauce)
1/2 tsp baking powder
6 **Brazil nuts**, shelled
3 medium **carrots**, peeled and grated
4 dried **apricots**, finely chopped
1 **egg**, beaten
a little olive oil
TO SERVE (OPTIONAL)
150g natural **yoghurt**
squeeze of **lemon** juice
small handful of chopped coriander

Put the chickpeas, onion, garlic, parsley, spices, baking powder and nuts in a blender and process briefly to a rough paste. Ideally there will still be a few chunks of Brazils. Tip the mixture into a bowl. If you prefer, you can break the nuts up with a pestle and mortar and add them at this stage (rather than earlier).

Add the grated carrots, chopped apricots and beaten egg and mix thoroughly. Form the mixture into 12 small balls and flatten them slightly.

Spray a non-stick pan with a little olive oil and place over a medium heat. Add the falafel and fry lightly until they're brown on both sides.

Meanwhile, if you are serving it, flavour the yoghurt with lemon juice and coriander to taste. Serve the falafel warm, with the yoghurt.

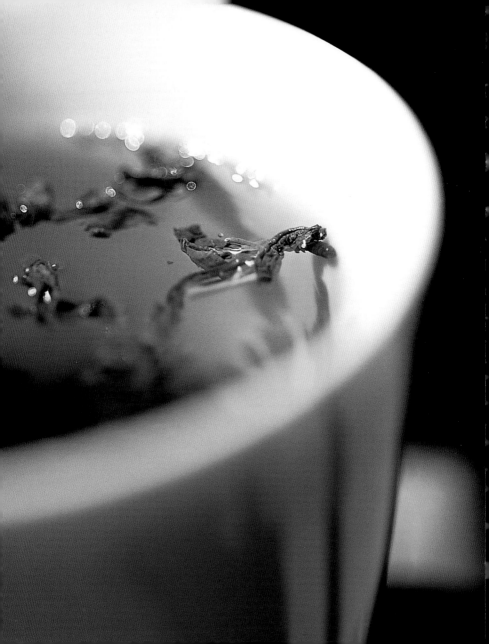

green tea

The leaves for this delicate drink come from the same plant as black tea but they are lightly steamed when freshly cut, rather than left to dry out and turn black, so more of the goodness is preserved. There are several antioxidant chemicals called flavonoids in green tea that make it so beneficial, but the most effective is thought to be one called epigallocatechin gallate. Oxidants are an inevitable part of life, our bodies even produce them, but pollution, the sun, smoking, smoky atmospheres and fried foods expose us to even more. An excess of oxidants has been linked to chronic conditions such as heart disease and cancer, as well as accelerated ageing. Given that green tea can contain about eight times as much antioxidant power as black tea, a couple of cups a day is certain to offer some protection. Gut-wise, the tannins in tea can help stop diarrhoea. Remember though, that green tea does contain some caffeine, which can irritate the gut, stimulate the nervous system and make you restless.

poached figs

USE EITHER LOOSE LEAVES OR A TEABAG TO MAKE THE GREEN TEA FOR THIS
LOVELY, LIGHT DESSERT, WHICH CAN ALSO BE SERVED AS A SIDE DISH TO GRILLED
OR ROASTED MEAT.

1 mugful of **green tea**
2 tbsp **honey**
6 **thyme** sprigs, plus extra
   sprigs to serve
100ml Marsala wine
½ **lemon**, sliced (pips
   removed)
8 fresh, ripe figs, washed
   and cut in half
natural **yoghurt**, to serve

In a large saucepan, combine the green tea, honey, thyme and wine. Bring to the boil, lower the heat and add the lemon slices. Stir constantly until the honey is completely dissolved.

Halve the figs vertically, add them to the green tea solution and poach for about 2 minutes on each side. Remove the figs with a slotted spoon and place in serving bowls.

Boil the liquid in the pan until it is syrupy. Drizzle the syrup all over the figs and top each portion with a slice of lemon and some thyme. Serve with natural yoghurt or cream.

green tea refresher

THIS IS A WONDERFUL DRINK ON A HOT SUMMER DAY. YOU CAN USE OTHER TYPES
OF FRUIT JUICE — FRESHLY SQUEEZED GRAPEFRUIT IS PARTICULARLY TANGY.

3 mugfuls of freshly made
green tea
*5cm piece fresh root **ginger**,*
peeled and grated
small bunch of mint leaves
*1 mugful of **pineapple** juice*
lots of ice cubes

Combine the freshly made green tea with the
ginger and half the mint in a large jug and set
aside to cool.

Add the rest of the mint, the pineapple juice
and the ice cubes just before serving and stir well.

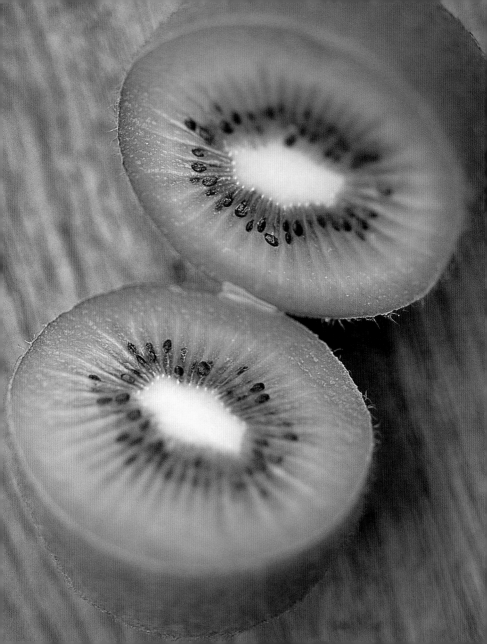

kiwi fruit

New Zealanders renamed the Chinese gooseberry in the 1950s as a marketing strategy, hence the name 'kiwi fruit'. Still, it beats the original French name of *souris vegetale* or 'vegetable mouse'. Whatever you call them, kiwi fruit are, like most foods in this section, loaded with antioxidants, including a member of the carotene family, lutein, as well as vitamins C and E. Scientists have found that eating two or three kiwi fruit a day helps reduce blood clotting (and therefore stroke) potential as well as blood fats. Kiwis are right up there with bananas on the potassium front, so they are good for balancing out your salt intake to keep your blood pressure right. Kiwis are also digestive aids, firstly because they are high in fibre that's useful for blood sugar control and for helping lower cholesterol. Secondly because they contain an enzyme called actinidin, which actually helps digest proteins in food – like the enzyme papain in papaya. Beware though, that some people, especially young children can have an allergic reaction to kiwi fruit, especially from its skin.

kiwi & figs with parma ham

I FIRST ATE THIS AT A FRIEND'S HOUSE IN THE SOUTH OF FRANCE — IT'S A
SURPRISINGLY WONDERFUL COMBINATION.

4 ripe **kiwi fruit,** peeled
4 ripe figs
8 thin slices of Parma ham
splash of balsamic vinegar
    (optional)
splash of olive oil (optional)

Slice the kiwi fruit in half lengthways and the figs into three from top to bottom. Arrange a fig and a kiwi on each plate, along with two slices of Parma ham.

I don't think there is any need for a dressing here, but if you like, drizzle with a little balsamic vinegar and a splash of olive oil.

pastel perfect kiwi

A DELICIOUS SMOOTHIE THAT CAN BE SHARP ON THE TONGUE IF THE FRUITS
AREN'T NICE AND RIPE, SO PICK YOUR MOMENT WELL.

½ **pineapple**, peeled, cored
   and roughly chopped
3 **kiwi fruit**, peeled
120ml **pineapple** juice

Put all the ingredients in a blender and whiz until smooth. Drink immediately.

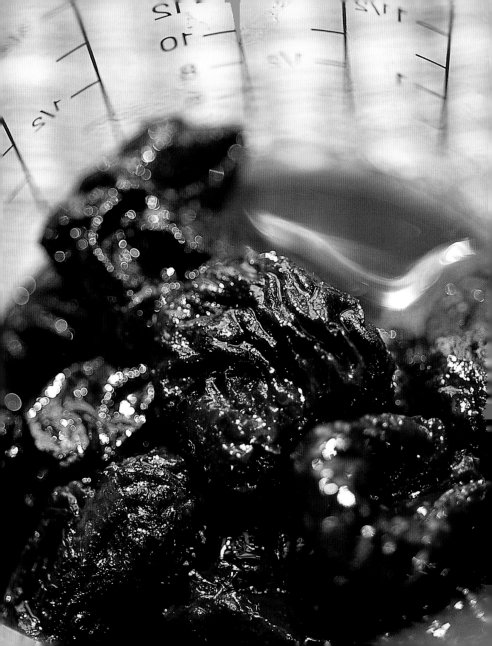

prunes

Of course, prunes have long been recognised as a very rich source of fibre that's good for keeping your bowel movements regular, but there is much more to them than that. Prunes are one of the top foods for total antioxidant power. These vital chemicals in foods are essential for keeping your skin clear, improving your detoxification, protecting you from disease and generally keeping the inevitable ageing process in check. So don't wait until your face looks like one to start eating prunes – even they won't reverse wrinkles. However, scientists have shown that your diet can affect how wrinkly your skin becomes with age. There's more – prunes are fat free and high in the important minerals potassium and iron. Remember that prunes are dried plums; the two words (the former French, the latter, Anglo-Saxon) were used interchangeably until recent times). So plump, fresh plums are also wonderfoods, just less so than prunes, weight for weight.

moroccan lamb

THIS IS AN ABSOLUTE FAVOURITE IN OUR HOME ON A WINTER'S NIGHT — WITH ALL THOSE AROMAS, YOU COULD BE IN MARRAKECH BUT FOR THE COLD OUTSIDE.

300g lean **lamb**
3 **garlic** cloves, crushed
1 tbsp harissa or chilli paste
juice of 1 **lemon**
freshly ground black pepper
small handful of mint,
    chopped
splash of olive oil
8 **shallots**, peeled
1 **cinnamon** stick
7 **cardamom** pods
2 tsp ground cumin
5 medium-large **tomatoes**,
    skinned and chopped
250g **chickpeas** (cooked or
    canned and drained)
10–12 **prunes**
about 600ml water
small handful of coriander
    leaves, chopped

Cut the lamb into bite-sized cubes. In a bowl, mix the garlic with the harissa, lemon juice, some pepper and half the mint. Add the lamb, toss to coat and leave to marinate while you prepare the other ingredients.

Heat a splash of olive oil in a large saucepan, then add the shallots with the spices and cook, stirring, for a minute or two. Add the lamb, together with its marinade, and stir well for a few minutes until it is lightly browned all over. Add the tomatoes, chickpeas and prunes, plus the water. Stir well, cover and leave to simmer for about an hour until the lamb is tender.

Add the remaining mint and coriander just before serving. Eat with brown rice or cous cous.

drunken prunes

EVEN PEOPLE WHO SAY THEY DON'T LIKE PRUNES LOVE THIS RICH DESSERT.

20–24 **prunes**
100ml **apple** juice
100ml water
50ml brandy
2.5cm piece fresh root
   ginger, peeled and sliced
finely pared zest of
   1 **orange**
10–12 **almonds**, shelled
TO SERVE
150g natural **yoghurt**
½ tsp vanilla extract, or
   to taste

Put the prunes in a saucepan and add the apple juice, water, brandy, ginger and orange zest. Bring to the boil, then immediately turn the heat down to a simmer. Cook, uncovered, for 15–20 minutes.

Meanwhile, toast the almonds for a few minutes under a hot grill and then roughly crush them, using a pestle and mortar or small food processor. Mix the yoghurt with the vanilla extract.

Using a slotted spoon, divide the prunes among four bowls. Top with a dollop of yoghurt and drizzle with some of the cooking liquor. Sprinkle with the crushed almonds and serve.

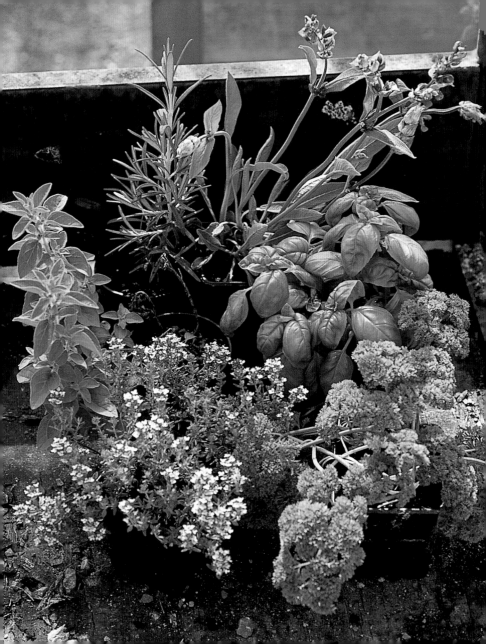

mediterranean
herbs

The scent of fresh, wild thyme being crushed under my feet on Maltese cliff tops is a strong childhood memory, but the aroma is just part of the story. Mediterranean herbs – thyme, sage, parsley, oregano, basil and rosemary – are brimming with health benefits that have been recognised for ages. Herbs were used to help preserve foods, to protect them from microbial contamination, and now research has shown that they protect us too. All, but especially oregano, contain chemicals that kill infectious microbes. Thymol, an oil in thyme leaves, is powerfully antiseptic and good for coughs and chest infections. It also helps protect the fats found in cell membranes, particularly the brain and heart, from oxidant damage and therefore rapid ageing. Eugenol and apigenin, found in basil, parsley and rosemary, have anti-inflammatory properties that can help with conditions such as arthritis, asthma and bowel inflammation. A cup of fresh sage and rosemary tea is wonderful for digestion or even a cough.

herby sweet oven chips

WHO NEEDS NORMAL CHIPS WHEN YOU CAN HAVE THESE SWEET POTATO CHIPS?
THEY GO WELL WITH ANY MAIN COURSE, OR YOU CAN HAVE THEM AS A STARTER
WITH DIPS, SUCH AS APRICOT SALSA (PAGE 175) OR AVOCADO CREAM (PAGE 127).

*4 medium **sweet potatoes**,*
scrubbed
*several **oregano** sprigs*
*several **thyme** sprigs*
good splash of olive oil
freshly ground black pepper

Preheat the oven to 180°C/Gas 4. Cut the sweet potatoes lengthways into chunky, wedge-shaped pieces. Put them in a baking dish with the herbs and olive oil. Season with pepper and toss well. Bake for about 30 minutes until tender – a skewer or sharp knife will slide through easily. Drain on kitchen paper and serve.

white bean mash

MY FRIEND JANET KIPLING MADE THESE FOR ME ONE WINTER'S EVENING. YOU CAN
ACTUALLY LEAVE THESE COOKED BEANS UNMASHED IF YOU PREFER, EATING THEM
EITHER HOT OR COOL AS A SALAD.

splash of olive oil
*1 large **onion**, peeled and*
*   chopped*
*2–3 **rosemary** sprigs*
*4–6 **sage** leaves*
*500g butter **beans** or*
*   haricot **beans** (cooked or*
*   canned and drained)*
*2 **garlic** cloves, peeled and*
*   finely chopped*
150ml water
pinch of sea salt
freshly ground black pepper
1 tsp whole grain mustard
*1 tbsp chopped **parsley***

Heat the olive oil in a large saucepan. Add the
onion, with the rosemary and sage, and cook until
softened but don't let it brown. Toss in the beans,
then add the garlic, water, salt and pepper. Leave
to simmer gently for about 20 minutes. Take out
the woody rosemary stems. (I leave the herb
leaves in for colour.)

Mash the bean mixture well, adding the
mustard and parsley as you do so. Serve with a
tomato salad, or as a side dish to meat or fish.

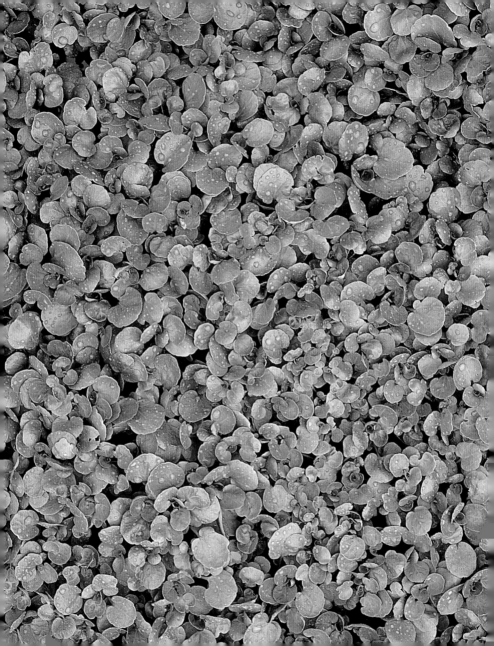

watercress

This peppery green has been eaten since ancient times and even used as a remedy for catarrh, bronchitis and scurvy. It is, these days, an under-rated food, although it's packed with those all-important antioxidants including members of the carotene family, lutein and zeaxanthin, as well as the powerful anti-inflammatory quercetin. Weight for weight, it is as rich as oranges in vitamin C, which is essential for keeping our skin regenerating well, our liver healthy and our defences strong. With ageing from oxidant damage, we're not just talking about visible external wrinkles, but also the health of our internal organs — essential for a long, healthy life. In common with other members of the cruciferous family (like broccoli and cabbage) watercress contains glucosinolates, which help the liver's detoxification capacity. One type in particular, phenylethyl isothiocyanate, has been shown to have anti-cancer properties. Watercress also helps the release of bile from the gall bladder, which is important for fat digestion and works as a natural laxative.

monkfish with watercress sauce

YOU CAN USE ANY FISH FOR THIS DISH, BUT PEPPERY WATERCRESS COMPLEMENTS
WHITE FISH PARTICULARLY WELL.

1 tbsp **sunflower seeds**
1 tbsp olive oil
4 **shallots**, peeled and finely
    diced
1 **garlic** clove, peeled and
    crushed
4 portions of **monkfish** or
    other white **fish** fillet,
    each about 150g
juice of 1–2 **lemons**
3–4 handfuls of **watercress**,
    washed and roughly
    chopped
freshly ground black pepper
2 tbsp soured cream

In a large, dry frying pan over a medium heat, toss
the sunflower seeds until they are golden. Then
add the olive oil and soften the shallots and garlic
over a low heat until they turn opaque.

Add the fish portions and cook gently for about
2 minutes, then turn and cook the other side for a
couple of minutes. Sprinkle with the lemon juice
then add the watercress to the pan, stirring it
around so it wilts. Season with pepper. Turn the
fish again and cook for another 2 minutes or until
cooked through; it will need around 8 minutes in
total, depending on the thickness of the fillets.

Add the soured cream and heat gently, stirring
it into the watercress around the fish. Serve the
fish topped with the sauce.

scrambled eggs with watercress

CREAMY SOFT EGGS AND SHARP, FRESH-TASTING WATERCRESS IS A WONDERFUL
COMBINATION. FOR A RICHER, MORE DECADENT VERSION, SERVE IT WITH A COUPLE
OF SLICES OF SMOKED SALMON AND A SPRINKLING OF FRESHLY CHOPPED DILL.

*6 **eggs***
freshly ground black pepper
pinch of salt
*dash of milk or **soya** milk*
1 tsp butter
*2 handfuls of **watercress**,*
washed and roughly
chopped
whole grain rye toast,
lightly buttered, to serve

Beat the eggs in a bowl with pepper, salt and a dash of milk.

Heat the butter in a saucepan, add the eggs and stir constantly over a very low heat until they are the texture you like – the secret lies in cooking them slowly. A minute or so before they are ready, stir in the watercress so it wilts.

Serve the lot on top of hot, lightly buttered whole grain rye toast.

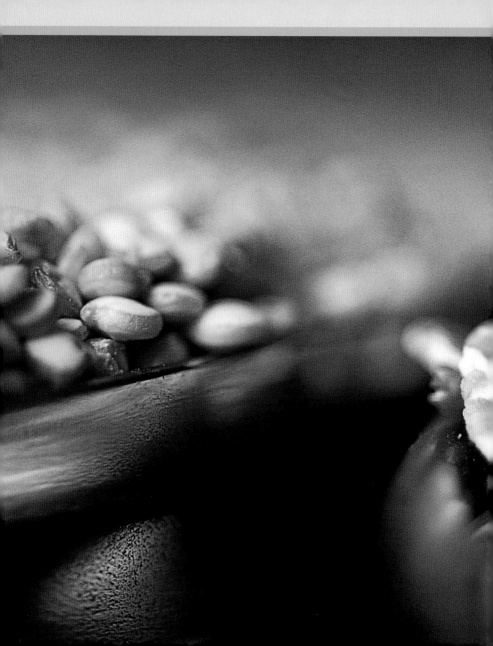

mind

The wonderfoods in this section contain nutrients that help to balance out moods, to calm you down when you are anxious and to get a good night's sleep. Even if you are someone who relies on alcohol or drugs to help you relax, these foods can help you chill out further. Eaten as part of a varied intake, they could even help you to reduce your dependence on ultimately detrimental short-term solutions.

Certain foods contain natural substances that help quieten down the nervous system, such as the gramine in oats. The minerals, calcium and magnesium, work in tandem to balance the nervous system and muscle contraction-relaxation. Both sunflower and sesame seeds are good sources of these two minerals, while yoghurt provides calcium. Just working on calming the nervous system, however, is not the only answer. It's also important to support the body's stress response by keeping the adrenal glands well nourished with nutrients such as pantothenic acid, B5, found in seeds and whole grains.

Keeping blood sugar levels well balanced is an important part of reducing anxiety, restful sleep and even moods. Having three meals a day, plus two snacks if necessary, can help this, by ensuring that the body does not go for too long without fuel. Eating a protein-rich food such as yoghurt, chicken or eggs means that the release of energy from the meal is sustained rather than sudden. These two strategies alone are a good start in reducing anxiety and low moods; they also put you in a position where you are less likely to need the lift or the downer from sugar, caffeine, cigarettes, drugs or booze.

One of the chemicals that the body produces naturally for good moods is the neurotransmitter (nerve messenger molecule), serotonin. The amino acid, tryptophan – found in chicken, yoghurt and seeds, amongst other foods – is one of the raw ingredients for making serotonin. Others are B vitamins and zinc, found in the same foods and whole grains. In order for serotonin to, in effect, transmit a message from one cell to the next, the gateway to the cell – its membrane – needs to be in good shape. Healthy membranes incorporate important fats such as those derived from seeds and phosphatidylcholine, a substance derived from the choline in eggs.

There is more, of course, to keeping calm and happy than keeping your cells on good form, serotonin production and even blood sugar levels. If patches of stress seem to stretch on for ever, assessing and dealing with what is going on in your life, your lifestyle and the way you react to events – with professional help if need be – is fundamental.

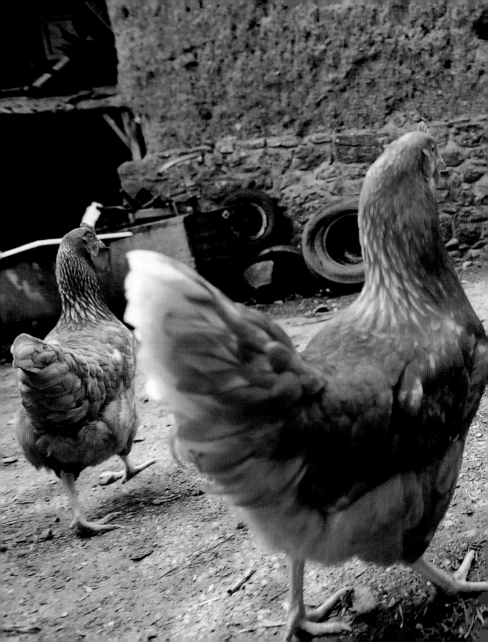

turkey & chicken

You don't need to wait for the festive season to have turkey on the table, as portions are now readily available. Skinless turkey breast is about the leanest meat there is, so it's an excellent source of protein – one portion giving you as much as half your daily need. Organic, free-range chicken is good too and both meats contain the amino acid, tryptophan. The body can convert tryptophan into serotonin, in effect, a 'happy hormone' that also helps you feel relaxed. Turkey and chicken provide doses of B vitamins – needed to make energy, to respond to stress and also to actually turn tryptophan into serotonin. These lean meats are rich in the mineral zinc, which has countless uses in the body; studies have shown many people with depression are low in zinc. Having protein food, such as turkey or chicken, makes a meal more satisfying for longer, which in turn helps keep energy, moods and concentration more even. The majority of chickens and turkeys are reared very intensively, so buy organic.

lemongrass turkey skewers

MY FRIEND, THE CHEF, ALAN WICHERT MAKES THIS WONDERFUL DISH DURING THE
HEALTHY FITNESS HOLIDAYS WE WORK AT TOGETHER IN MARRAKECH. IT ALWAYS
GOES DOWN A STORM WITH GUESTS. IF YOU CAN'T FIND LEMONGRASS YOU CAN
USE METAL OR WOODEN SKEWERS (SOAKING THE LATTER BEFORE COOKING).

juice of 1 **lime**
juice of ½ **orange**
1 tsp harissa paste
1 tsp cumin seeds
1 tsp fennel seeds
1 tbsp olive oil
2 large, skinless **turkey**
breasts
8 lemongrass stalks
1 courgette, sliced into
1cm discs
1 red **pepper***, cored,*
deseeded and cut into
squares
8 shiitake **mushrooms***, cut*
in half
½ **pineapple***, peeled, cored*
and cubed

In a large bowl, mix together the lime juice, orange juice, harissa, cumin seeds, fennel seeds and olive oil. Cut the turkey into bite-sized chunks, add to the bowl and toss well. Cover and leave to marinate in a cool place, ideally for at least 2 hours.

Thread the turkey pieces on to the lemongrass 'skewers', alternating with the courgette, red pepper, mushrooms and pineapple. Preheat the grill, barbecue or a griddle pan (oiling this lightly) and cook the skewers, turning occasionally, for about 10 minutes until evenly coloured and the turkey is cooked through.

Serve the skewers with Mango & pineapple salsa (page 134) and brown rice.

crusted roasted chicken

A TASTY CRUST FLAVOURS SKINLESS CHICKEN THIGHS AND HELPS TO KEEP THEM
MOIST DURING BAKING.

1 red **onion**, peeled and
    quartered
1 **garlic** clove, peeled
1 tbsp chopped lemon
    thyme
1 tsp balsamic vinegar
2 tbsp Parmesan cheese,
    freshly grated
1 tbsp olive oil
4 tbsp **sunflower seeds**
8 **chicken** thighs, skin
    removed

Preheat the oven to 180°C/Gas 4. Using a pestle
and mortar, pound the onion, garlic, lemon thyme,
balsamic vinegar, Parmesan and olive oil together.
Add the sunflower seeds and work to a rough
paste, adding a spoonful of water if necessary.

Lay the chicken pieces in an ovenproof dish
and smother them generously with the crust
mixture. Pour a little water into the dish, just
enough to cover the bottom, and bake for about
30 minutes until the chicken is cooked through.

Delicious with brown rice or buckwheat and
Green spice stir-fry (page 95) or steamed broccoli.

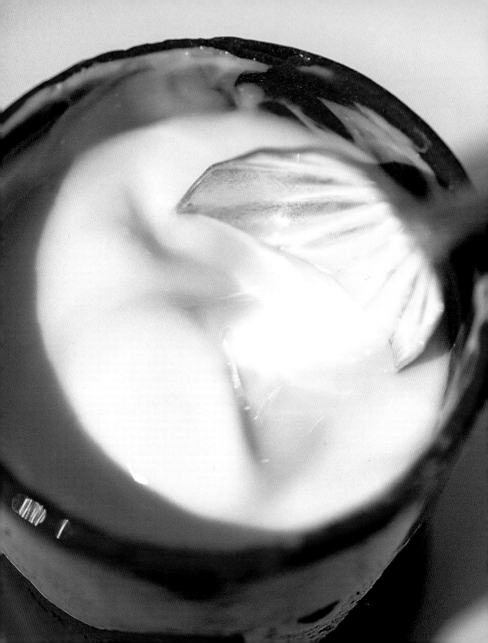

yoghurt

Ever since cows were first domesticated, humans have been eating fermented milk, and its benefits have long been recognised. Yoghurt is made by adding lactobacillus and bifidobacteria cultures to milk but it's important to buy 'live' yoghurts as some are pasteurised after the culture is added, killing it off. Live bacteria are well-known beneficial inhabitants of our digestive tracts as they help maintain the correct acidity, enhance immunity and aid digestion. Lactobacillus and bifidobacteria have also been shown to help lower cholesterol levels. Yoghurt is a good protein food, particularly for vegetarians. It contains tryptophan, the precursor of serotonin, the mood-booster. Some people who react badly to milk products are fine with yoghurt because bacteria ferment it by eating the milk sugar (lactose), making it more digestible. Like all milk products, yoghurt is a rich source of calcium, which is essential for healthy bones but also for muscles to work properly, and for nerves to fire their messages efficiently.

salmon with seaweed sauce

ALTHOUGH I'VE USED SALMON HERE, YOU CAN COOK ANY FISH YOU FANCY TO GO
WITH THIS SAUCE.

6 tbsp natural **yoghurt**
1cm piece fresh root **ginger**,
    peeled and grated
1 **garlic** clove, peeled and
    grated
grated zest and juice of
    1 **lime**
2 tbsp **sesame** oil
½ tsp cayenne pepper
4 **salmon** (or other **fish**)
    steaks, each about 175g
2 tbsp dried **seaweed**, such
    as arame or hijiki

Mix the yoghurt, ginger, garlic, lime zest and juice, sesame oil and cayenne together in a shallow bowl. Add the fish and swish it around in the mixture to coat it well. Set aside to marinate for about 20 minutes.

Meanwhile, put the seaweed in a mug and pour over just enough boiling water to cover it. Leave to steep for 4–5 minutes.

Put the salmon steaks and marinade in a large frying pan over a medium heat, together with the seaweed and its water. Lower the heat when the liquid start to bubble and cook for 10–15 minutes or until the fish steaks are cooked, turning them halfway through.

Accompany with steamed or stir-fried kale and brown rice.

berry fool

THIS DESSERT IS SO HEALTHY THAT YOU CAN GET AWAY WITH HAVING A BUTTERY, CRUMBLY SHORTBREAD TO ACCOMPANY IT! USE THICK YOGHURT AND THE FOOL WON'T BE TOO RUNNY. WHEN FRESH BERRIES ARE OUT OF SEASON IT'S FINE TO USE FROZEN ONES.

*400g mixed **berries**, such as raspberries, blueberries and strawberries*
*250g thick natural **yoghurt** (ideally Greek)*
2 tsp caster sugar or alternative equivalent (see page 10)

Put the ingredients into a blender, saving a few whole berries for serving, and whiz until evenly blended. Divide among individual pots and top each serving with a couple of berries.

Serve shortbread biscuits or small meringues on the side.

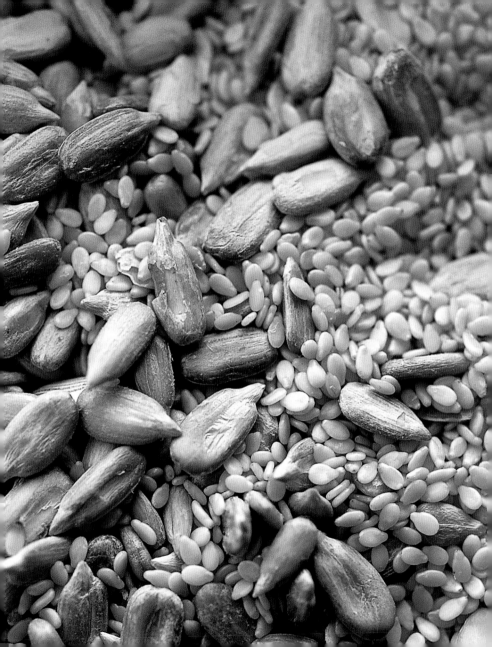

sunflower &
sesame seeds

These little seeds are powerhouses of nutrients: sunflower seeds from the studded centres of the vivid yellow flowers and tiny sesame seeds, which in ancient India were a symbol of immortality. Both seeds are good sources of vitamin E, plus omega 6 and monounsaturated fats, which all help minimise heart disease as well as boost the elasticity of skin. They are also rich in calcium and magnesium, needed for relaxation and contraction of muscles (including the heart) and bone health. Magnesium is required for each cell to produce energy, yet it is also considered the 'calming' mineral. The zinc and selenium in sunflower and sesame seeds (as well sesamol and other chemicals) are important antioxidants. Low levels of zinc are associated with poor immunity, infertility, bad skin and depression. The vitamin B5 in the seeds is essential for a healthy response to stress. Sesame seeds, because of their size, are often left undigested, which means that the nutrient content is missed. When chewed thoroughly though, or used as a paste (tahini) you can get their full benefits.

sunny salad

EVEN IF YOU CAN'T GET HOLD OF ANY OF THE FLOWERS FOR THIS, IT'S STILL A COLOURFUL SALAD, BRIMMING WITH GOODNESS. AND IF YOU'VE NEVER TASTED PROPER, COLD-PRESSED SUNFLOWER OIL BEFORE, YOU WON'T RECOGNISE ITS GORGEOUSLY NUTTY AND RICH FLAVOUR. BORAGE IS KNOWN AS A CALMING HERB.

1 yellow **pepper**, cored, deseeded and chopped
handful of **watercress** leaves
½ red-leaved lettuce, such as lollo rosso
selection of nasturtium, borage and marigold flowers
2 spring **onions**, trimmed and sliced
1 tbsp **sunflower seeds**
1 tbsp cold-pressed **sunflower oil**
capful of cider vinegar

Toss all the ingredients together just before serving, as a side salad with a main dish such as Sesame-studded mackerel (opposite).

sesame-studded mackerel

I OFTEN COOK MACKEREL THIS WAY, BUT YOU COULD CHOOSE ANY FISH YOU LIKE.

4 tbsp **sesame seeds**
2 tbsp chopped chives
4 **mackerel** fillets
a little **sesame** oil
1 **lime**, cut into wedges,
   to serve

Mix the sesame seeds and chives together on a large plate and then press both sides of the fish fillets on to them, so that the seeds as well as the chives adhere.

Heat a griddle or frying pan and add a little sesame oil. Cook the fish for 2–3 minutes each side, depending on the thickness of the fillets.

Serve with lime wedges and accompany with soba noodles and a salad or stir-fried spinach.

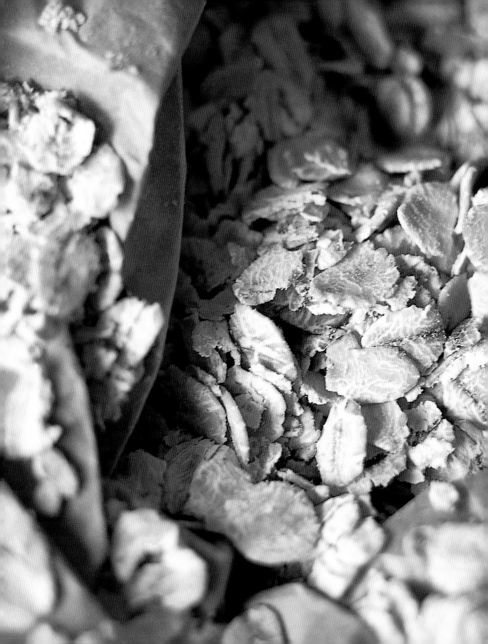

oats

Good, old-fashioned oats are a remarkably versatile grain with wide-ranging health properties. In addition to being a good source of carbohydrates, they are high in both soluble and insoluble fibre. This means they are digested slowly and don't raise blood sugar levels dramatically. Consequently, oats will keep both mood and energy levels even for a while after they are eaten – making them an ideal breakfast food. The fibre contributes to a healthy gut, not just keeping you regular but also binding to waste products. Studies have shown that oats can also help lower cholesterol. Herbalists recommend oat extracts to help calm anxiety and depression, which is probably why oat tincture has been recommended for people trying to quit smoking. Oats are loaded with B vitamins, vitamin E and important minerals such as iron and zinc. All of these are needed for a healthy nervous system, as well as much, much more. They are also one of the richest food sources of silicon, needed for healthy skin and bones. Use this versatile grain to make porridge, oaty snack bars or crumble toppings.

crunchy plum crumble

THIS A WONDERFUL VERSION OF THE TRADITIONAL ENGLISH DESSERT. YOU CAN
REPLACE THE PLUMS WITH APPLES, RHUBARB OR BERRIES IF YOU LIKE.

500g **muesli**
1 tsp ground **cinnamon**
2 tbsp **pumpkin seeds**
10 **walnuts**, shelled and
    broken into pieces
40g butter, in pieces
800g **plums**, halved and
    stoned
4–5 star anise
1 tbsp brown sugar
5 tbsp water
TO SERVE
150g natural **yoghurt**
½ tsp vanilla extract, or
    to taste

Preheat the oven to 180°C/Gas 4. Combine the
muesli, cinnamon, pumpkin seeds and walnuts in
a large mixing bowl. Add the butter and rub in
using your fingertips until there are no lumps of
butter left. Alternatively, you can melt the butter
and mix it in that way.

Lay the plums and star anise in a baking dish
and sprinkle with the sugar and water. Spoon the
crumble mixture over the top of the plums, so that
they are well covered. Bake the crumble for about
40 minutes or until the plums are soft when
tested with a skewer.

Mix some natural yoghurt with a little vanilla
extract to serve on the side, or, more indulgently,
have vanilla ice cream or custard.

fruity porridge

THERE'S NO BETTER START TO THE DAY THAN A BOWL OF HOT PORRIDGE. ADDING FRUIT GIVES AN UNUSUAL TEXTURE AND SWEETNESS, THOUGH IT CAN BE ADDED AFTER YOU'VE COOKED THE PORRIDGE IF YOU PREFER. YOU COULD REPLACE THE APPLE OR PEAR WITH 2–3 TBSP STEWED RHUBARB OR A FEW STEWED PLUMS. SERVES 2

5 tbsp porridge **oats**
about 200ml milk or **soya milk**
1 **apple** or **pear**, grated
1 tsp **honey** or maple syrup
2 tbsp **High five mix** (page 154)

Put the oats in a saucepan, add water to cover and stir with a wooden spoon over a low heat. As the oats begin to absorb the water, slowly start to add the milk, stirring all the time. Add the fruit. Each time the porridge starts to thicken, add a little more milk to keep it slightly runny.

When the oats are cooked – this should take about 5 minutes – stir in the honey or maple syrup, top with High five mix and serve.

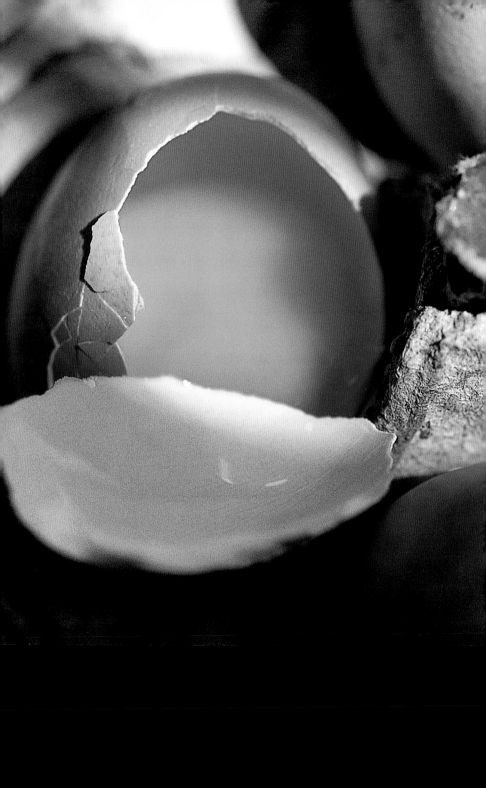

egg

Eggs get a bad press due to their cholesterol content, but as an excellent source of protein, vitamins, minerals and, most interestingly, unsaturated fats, they are a wonderfood in a neat shell. Of the 5g of fat in an egg, most is monounsaturated (like in olive oil), which actually helps lower the risk of heart disease. Anyway, we need some cholesterol for a healthy brain and for making the sex and stress hormones. Egg yolk is the richest known source of choline, which helps keep cholesterol fluid, preventing it from clogging up arteries. Choline also makes up cell membranes, helps the body process fats and converts to acetylcholine, an important memory molecule in the brain. The yolk's rich colour comes from beneficial antioxidants, lutein and zeaxanthin. Eggs are a great source of iron, zinc and selenium, plus A and B vitamins. The truth is an egg is as nutritious as the chicken that laid it – so buy only organic or free-range and an egg a day could help keep the doctor away.

asparagus & sunchoke tortilla

IF YOU CAN'T GET HOLD OF JERUSALEM ARTICHOKES, USE BABY NEW POTATOES FOR THIS SPANISH-STYLE OMELETTE. YOU'LL NEED A FRYING PAN THAT'S SUITABLE TO USE BRIEFLY UNDER THE GRILL.

8 *Jerusalem artichokes*, scrubbed
juice of ¹/₂ **lemon**
8 **eggs**
4–6 **basil** leaves, torn
freshly ground black pepper
pinch of fine sea salt
splash of olive oil
handful of **spinach** leaves, roughly chopped
8 thin **asparagus** spears, cut into pieces
2 medium **tomatoes**, sliced

Boil the Jerusalem artichokes in water to cover with the lemon juice until they feel tender when pierced with a skewer, about 15 minutes. Drain and allow to cool, then slice thickly.

Beat the eggs with the basil and seasoning. Preheat the grill.

Heat the olive oil in a large frying pan and add the egg mixture. Scatter the spinach, asparagus, artichokes and tomatoes evenly over the egg. Cook the tortilla for about 3 minutes on the hob (don't stir it) then under a grill for a minute or two until it's golden brown all over.

Serve the tortilla cut into wedges, with a Wonderfoods green salad (page 111).

broccoli polenta flan

POLENTA FORMS THE BASE FOR THIS 'FLAN', RATHER THAN THE USUAL PASTRY.
YOU COULD USE PRETTY MUCH ANY CHEESE YOU'VE GOT IN THE FRIDGE.

500ml vegetable or chicken
    stock
150g 'instant' polenta or
    cornmeal
2 tbsp freshly grated
    Parmesan cheese
walnut-sized knob of butter
a little olive oil

3 eggs

250ml milk
1/2 tsp mustard powder
1/2 tsp freshly grated nutmeg
freshly ground black pepper
pinch of fine sea salt
3 spring **onions**, trimmed
    and finely sliced
100g **broccoli**, cut into very
    small florets
50g Gruyère or strong
    Cheddar cheese, grated

Preheat the oven to 180°C/Gas 4. Bring the stock to the boil in a large saucepan. Turn down the heat and slowly add the polenta, whisking constantly to avoid it becoming lumpy. Add the Parmesan and butter as you continue to whisk. Cook the polenta, stirring regularly, until it is very thick and comes away from the sides of the pan easily, about 10 minutes.

Smear the bottom of a 23cm flan dish with olive oil, pour in the polenta and bake it in the oven for 30 minutes while you prepare the filling.

In a bowl, beat the eggs, milk, mustard, nutmeg, pepper and salt together. Scatter the spring onions, broccoli florets and half of the Gruyère evenly over the polenta base. Carefully pour the egg mixture over and sprinkle with the rest of the cheese. Bake for about 30 minutes until the egg is set.

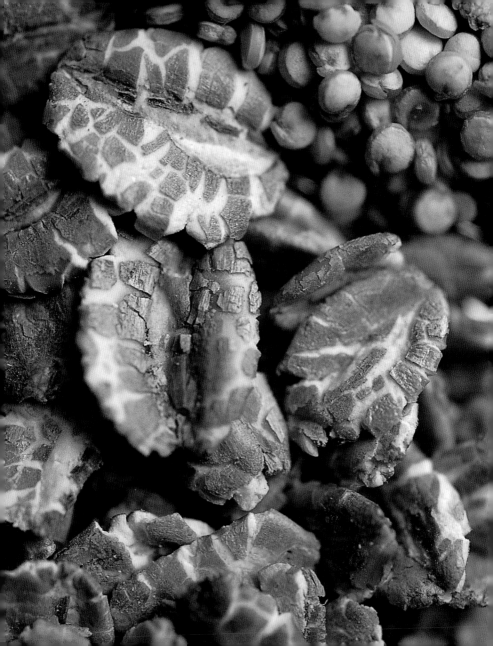

quinoa & rye

When the Spanish conquered Latin America, they forbade the cultivation of quinoa, realising what a fortifying, revered food it was. Pronounced *keen-wa* in its native land, it is known as the 'mother grain', indicating its significance – nutritionally and spiritually. When cooked, part of it separates, giving each grain a small halo! Quinoa contains significantly more protein than other grain foods and has the full range of essential amino acids. It also provides a spectrum of B vitamins, including B5, which is essential for the adrenal glands to mount a healthy stress response. Probably because of its hardy nature, rye is most popular in the coldest parts of Europe. It is particularly high in non-cellulose polysaccharides (fibre), which bind well with water, leaving you feeling more satisfied for longer after eating. It's also helpful for those managing their blood sugar balance, including diabetics. Rye is rich in antioxidants called phenolics and plant lignans, which protect the body from cancer and heart disease. Some lignans can help reduce the uncomfortable symptoms linked to the menopause.

fish stew with quinoa

THIS IS A VERY LIGHT, BROTHY STEW WITH A SUBTLE BLEND OF FLAVOURS. YOU CAN USE ANY SEAFOOD YOU FANCY, THOUGH FIRM-TEXTURED WHITE FISH AND A MIX OF SHELLFISH — PRAWNS, MUSSELS, CLAMS ETC. — WORKS BEST.

a little olive oil
1 small **onion**, peeled and finely diced
3 **garlic** cloves, peeled and crushed
$^{1}/_{2}$ tsp cayenne pepper
$^{1}/_{2}$ tsp ground **turmeric**
$^{1}/_{2}$ tsp smoked paprika
1 green **pepper**, cored, deseeded and chopped
4 medium **tomatoes**, skinned and chopped
2 tbsp capers
generous splash of white wine
300ml vegetable or fish stock
200g filleted **fish**, such as monkfish or chunky cod
about 8 raw prawns, shelled
about 8 mussels, cleaned
2 tbsp chopped **parsley**
FOR THE QUINOA
mugful of **quinoa**
2 mugfuls of water

Heat the olive oil in a large pan and soften the onion and garlic together with the spices over a low heat. Then add the green pepper, tomatoes and capers and stir for 2 or 3 minutes. Pour in the wine and stock and bring to the boil, then cover and leave to simmer for about 20 minutes, stirring occasionally.

Meanwhile, cook the quinoa. Rinse it well, then put it into a pan with the water and bring to the boil. Cover, turn down the heat to a simmer and cook for about 15 minutes.

Cut the fish into bite-sized chunks and add them to the tomato broth. Cover and cook for about 2 minutes, then add the prawns and mussels. Continue to cook until the prawns turn pink and the mussels open. Serve sprinkled with the chopped parsley, on a pile of quinoa.

designer muesli

THIS HOMEMADE MUESLI TAKES SECONDS TO MAKE, ALL TO YOUR OWN
SPECIFICATIONS. GOOD HEALTH FOOD SHOPS SELL A RANGE OF OTHER GRAINS
THAT YOU CAN ADD TO THE MIX. AND OF COURSE, YOU CAN ADD ANY OTHER NUTS,
SEEDS OR DRIED FRUITS YOU LIKE. SOME GRAINS, SUCH AS QUINOA, ARE BEST
PUFFED AS THEY ARE INEDIBLE RAW.

200g **rye** flakes
200g **oat** flakes
200g barley flakes
100g puffed **quinoa**
2 tbsp **sunflower seeds**
2 tbsp **pumpkin seeds**
3 tbsp raisins
8 dried **apricots**, finely
    chopped
TO SERVE
milk, natural **yoghurt** or
    soya milk

Mix all the ingredients together in a large storage
container. Serve yourself a bowlful with fresh milk,
natural yoghurt or soya milk. Top with fresh fruit
if you like.

NOTE If you have a sensitive digestion, soak your
bowl of muesli overnight in milk or apple juice.

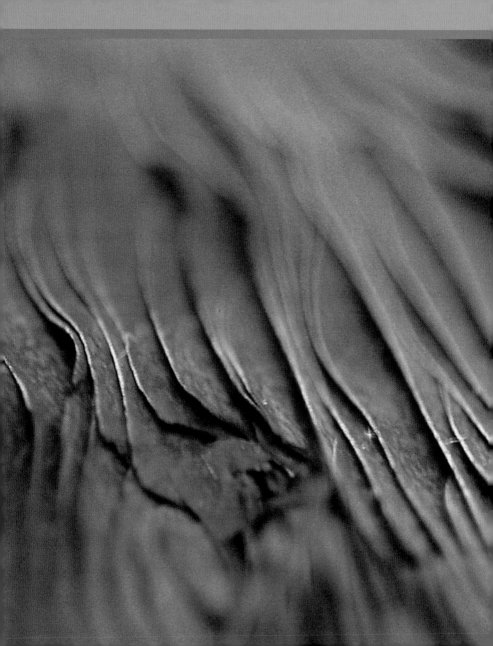

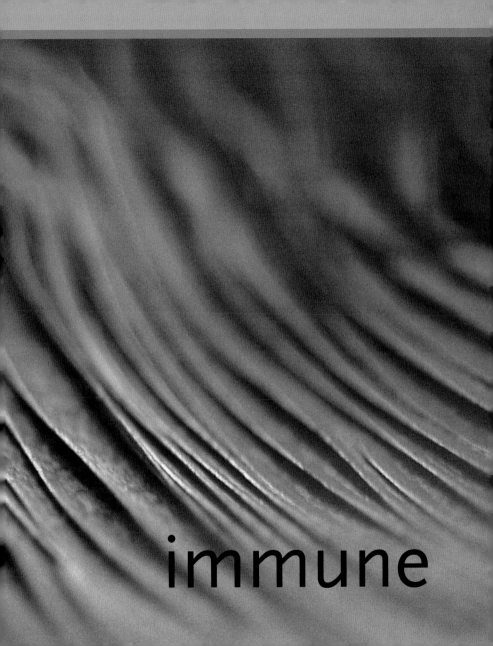

immune

Old-fashioned remedies are often just that because they've withstood the test of time and now scientists are showing that they make good modern sense too. Lemons for a cold, onions for a cough, shiitake mushrooms in Japan...are just some of the immune boosters you might find in an old wives' book of wonderfoods, and in mine too. Although, having tried it, I can't say that I would recommend homemade onion syrup, even if it did do the trick! The foods featured in this section of Wonderfoods are packed with vitamins, minerals and other naturally occurring substances that help our body's defences in the face of infection.

Our immune systems are remarkably intricate, consisting of countless sites and substances around the body that deal with potential pathogens – harmful, tiny organisms such as viruses, bacteria and fungi. Not only are there special defence chemicals in our skin and tears, but also all passages that open externally, such as our lungs and digestive tract, are lined with countless immune soldiers to neutralise would-be pathogens. If invaders manage to get through the first line of defences, further trouble lies in store for them in the form of immune cells that either patrol the body or sit waiting to pounce on anything that comes along. The body also produces special immune cells and substances to combat specific invaders; others detect and clear up suspect cells such as cancerous ones.

Not surprisingly, each person's immune system reacts at least slightly differently owing to our different genes and environments, even when we are exposed to the same pathogen. In some cases, one person may not even fall ill at all while another succumbs terribly to the same cold virus or tummy bug to which both were exposed. What makes the difference? The terrain into which the bug lands. Keep your body well up on nutrients that the immune system needs, such as those in these wonderfoods, and you'll be less likely to get ill. And if you do, you'll probably recover much more rapidly.

A good dose of immune wonderfoods is not all you'll need for keeping illness at bay. Stress is a big enemy of the immune system, as is too little sleep, not to mention the obvious factors like smoking and a high intake of alcohol. If, though, you have a diet that is high in immune wonderfoods, yet you still fall prey to infections regularly, you should work with a professional to see what could be pulling the rug out from beneath your body's defences.

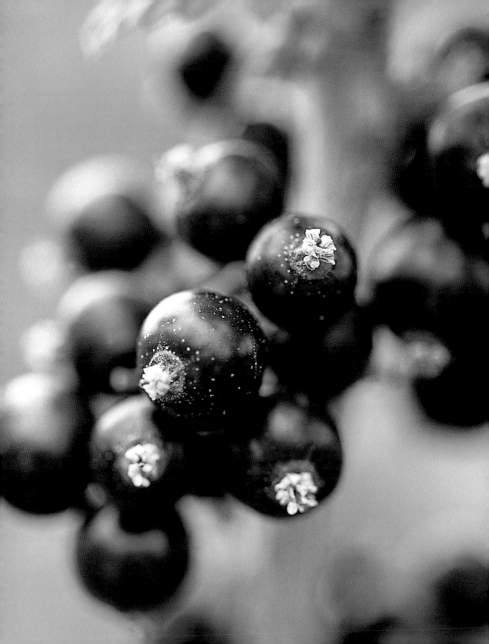

black**currants**

Historically, blackcurrants were grown for their medicinal properties and for turning to wine, or for making hot drinks to ease a sore throat. Because they are relatively tart, they are rarely eaten alone and these days, the closest many people get to them is in a sweetened cordial that shouts about its rich vitamin C content. Indeed, blackcurrants contain three times as much of this vital vitamin as oranges, weight for weight. Forget cordial though, with its high sugar content, and eat the fruit together with other foods that compensate for the sharpness. Blackcurrants are not just an extraordinary source of vitamin C, but also of its companion antioxidants, bioflavonoids, which are well known for boosting the body's defences. These compounds also help the condition of blood vessels, the skin and the stress response. In addition, the fibre and seeds in blackcurrants have long made them a good remedy for constipation, as they encourage the bowels to work smoothly.

blackcurrant smoothie

I LOVE THE CONTRAST OF SWEET, THICK BANANA AND TANGY BLACKCURRANTS
IN THIS REFRESHING DRINK. YOU CAN EVEN MAKE IT THROUGHOUT THE WINTER
USING BLACKCURRANTS CANNED IN NATURAL JUICE. CRUNCH WELL ON THE
BLACKCURRANT SEEDS AS THEY ARE FULL OF HEALTHY ESSENTIAL FATTY ACIDS.
SERVES 2

1 *banana*
2 heaped tbsp
 blackcurrants
4 tbsp natural *yoghurt*
200ml *apple* juice (or the
 juice from the
 blackcurrants, if using
 canned ones)

Whiz everything up in a blender, pour into glasses
and drink immediately.

NOTE This is enough for two good glasses full.

blackcurrant & apricot slice

THIS SLICE IS RELATIVELY IMPRESSIVE FOR THE EFFORT REQUIRED TO MAKE IT
AND IT'S DELICIOUS EATEN WARM, WITH VANILLA ICE CREAM. YOU COULD MAKE
INDIVIDUAL SQUARE OR TRIANGULAR PASTRIES IF YOU PREFER.

200g ready-made puff
    pastry
25g ground **almonds**
25g **almonds**, roughly
    chopped
1/2 tbsp butter, softened
2 tsp **walnut** or **hemp** oil,
    plus an extra 1 tsp to
    brush
1/2 tsp vanilla extract
1 tbsp **honey**
4 tbsp **blackcurrants**
4 **apricots**, halved, stoned
    and sliced

Preheat the oven to 200°C/Gas 6. Line a baking tray with greaseproof paper. Cut a rectangle of pastry about 25–30cm long and 10–12cm wide and lay it on the paper.

In a bowl, mix the ground and chopped almonds, butter, oil, vanilla and honey. Spread this mix over the pastry, leaving a 1cm margin all round. Lay the blackcurrants and apricots on top of the almond mixture. Brush the pastry edges with the hemp oil.

Bake for about 15 minutes until the pastry edges are puffed up and golden. Eat warm.

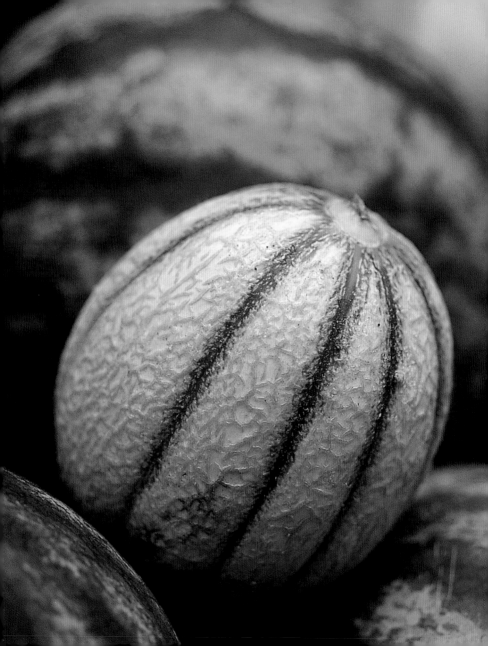

watermelon &
melon

Apart from the refreshing juiciness, the crunchy texture and the taste, watermelon has a lot to offer your health. For thousands of years watermelons have been valued in Africa and Asia (where aridity and polluted water are common) for their high content of sweet water. An impressive 90% of the flesh is water, so it is a refreshing cleanser and a diuretic. The red flesh is rich in powerful antioxidant nutrients, such as water soluble vitamin C and fat soluble lycopene and beta carotene – all important for helping your body's detoxification, fighting infections, protecting the eyes and lungs, slowing down ageing and countering inflammation. The seeds are loaded with yet more antioxidants such as zinc, selenium, vitamin E, plus essential fats, so crunch through them to get the full benefit. Pretty much all these nutrients contribute to fertility and sexual performance. Like watermelons, although not strictly related, melons are loaded with water and, particularly cantaloupe, with beta carotene.

watermelon & watercress salad

THIS HAS TO BE ONE OF THE MOST ZINGY, REFRESHING SALADS POSSIBLE BUT, TO MAKE IT MORE SO, YOU COULD ADD SOME GRAPEFRUIT SEGMENTS.

2 large slices of **watermelon**
2 large handfuls of
    watercress, trimmed
½ red **onion**, peeled and
    very finely sliced
1cm piece fresh root **ginger**,
    peeled and grated
2 tsp tamari or soy sauce
juice of 1 **lime**
4–6 **Brazil nuts**, roughly
    chopped
1 tbsp chopped coriander
    leaves

Cut the watermelon flesh away from the skin and chop the flesh into bite-sized pieces. Roughly chop the watercress and put it into a bowl with the watermelon and red onion.

Mix the ginger, tamari and lime juice together in a small bowl. Pour over the salad, add the nuts and coriander and toss to mix. Serve at once.

retro melon cocktail

BLENDING THE ENTIRE WATERMELON — SEEDS AND ALL — MEANS THAT YOU GET
THE MAXIMUM NUTRIENT VALUE, LET ALONE GREAT TASTE AND TEXTURE. AND IT'S
GREAT FOR HANGOVERS, OR, IF YOU LIKE, WITH A SHOT OF VODKA IN EACH GLASS.

$1/2$ **melon**, *such as*
cantaloupe
4 large chunks of
watermelon, *skin*
removed
3–4 mint leaves

Using a melon baller or teaspoon, scoop small
balls from the cantaloupe and set aside.

Put the watermelon flesh and seeds in a
blender with the mint and whiz until smooth. Pour
the watermelon smoothie into tall glasses and
serve it with the melon balls on cocktail sticks
balanced on the edge.

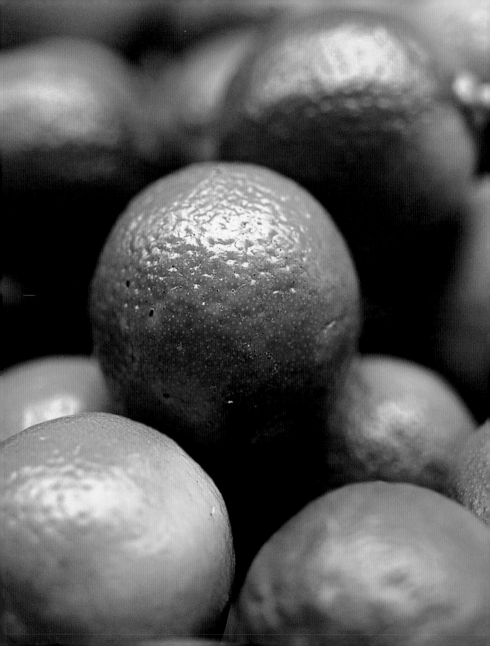

citrus fruit

As is so often the case with old wives' tales, there is more than a grain of truth that orange juice or a hot lemon drink will help you fight off a cold. Famously packed with the antioxidant vitamin C, citrus fruits give a good boost to the immune system. Vitamin C enhances the activity of white blood cells, increases the response of interferon (against viruses) and promotes antibodies. But there's a lot more to citrus fruits than that. The vitamin C is also important for the liver to work efficiently, and for healthy skin. The bitterness along with the limonene in lemons and limes stimulate the gall bladder, which helps the liver and digestion. Citrus fruits also contain bioflavonoids, such as rutin and quercitrin. These powerful antioxidants, in tandem with vitamin C, are particularly important for the health of blood vessels, so they have an impact on the cardiovascular system and help deter varicose veins. Compounds in citrus peel called polymethoxylated flavones have cholesterol-lowering effects.

tangy citrus cous cous

THIS MAKES A GOOD SUMMER SALAD FOR A PICNIC OR BARBECUE AND GOES WELL WITH GRILLED FISH OR PRAWNS.

200g cous cous
400ml freshly squeezed
    mixed **grapefruit** and
    orange juice
1 red **pepper**, cored,
    deseeded and chopped
1 courgette, trimmed and
    finely sliced
2 spring **onions**, trimmed
    and finely sliced
1 **garlic** clove, peeled and
    crushed
2 tbsp finely chopped mint
2 tbsp chopped coriander
2 tbsp olive oil
24 black olives

Put the cous cous in a bowl and pour on the fruit juice. Let the cous cous sit for about an hour, forking it through occasionally.

Prepare the other ingredients in the meantime. When the cous cous is soft, add all the other ingredients, toss to mix everything together well and serve.

prawns with lime chilli sauce

YOU COULD USE THIS MARINADE WITH ANY CHUNKY FISH OR SCALLOPS — EVEN THREAD SOME OF EACH ON TO SKEWERS.

1 tsp cumin seeds
grated zest and juice of
   1 **lime**
1 **garlic** clove, peeled and
   crushed
1 tbsp sweet chilli sauce
12 large raw prawns, shelled
   but with head and tails
   left on

In a small, dry frying pan, toast the cumin seeds over a medium heat until they are smoking slightly and giving off an aroma. Tip them into a bowl.

Add the lime zest and juice, the garlic and chilli sauce, stirring well. Add the prawns and swish them around to coat them in the mixture for a few minutes.

Preheat the grill, barbecue or a griddle pan (oiling it lightly). Cook the prawns quickly for a few minutes, turning them once or twice, until they just turn pink. Eat them immediately. Tangy citrus cous cous (opposite) is an ideal accompaniment.

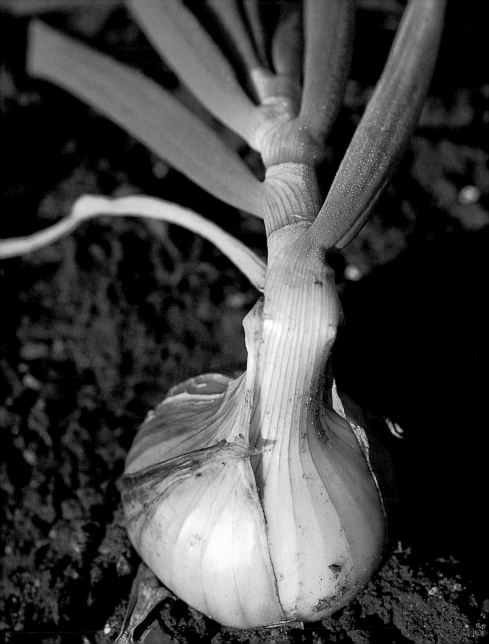

onion

I can't imagine cooking without onions, but in spiritual centres in India they are forbidden for their ability to light your inner fire. Arousal aside, onions are widely eaten all over the world and have been used for centuries for their medicinal properties. They contain allicin and other powerful, natural antibiotics that help fight off infections, including ones in the gut caused by parasites like worms. Allicin and another chemical, allylpropyldisulphide, help lower blood sugar. Onions also contain chemicals that relax the lung muscles and help the softening of mucus, so they are good for calming a cough. For the cardiovascular system, onions act as a diuretic, help to regulate blood pressure and help to prevent blood cells clumping. The sulphur in onions is a powerful detoxifier that boosts the liver, cleanses the gut, helps clear out toxic metals from the body (such as lead), and makes for a healthy skin. Onions also contain the antioxidant quercetin, which calms inflammation in the lungs (such as with asthma), helps protect against cancer and strengthens blood vessels.

sweet red onion polenta

THIS IS INSPIRED BY PISSALADIÈRE, A CARAMELISED ONION PIZZA SLICE FROM THE SOUTH OF FRANCE. YOU CAN LEAVE OUT THE ANCHOVIES IF YOU'RE VEGETARIAN OR NOT A FAN.

500ml vegetable or chicken stock
150g 'instant' polenta or cornmeal
2 tbsp freshly grated Parmesan cheese
1 tsp butter
1 tbsp olive oil, plus extra to brush
3 red **onions**, peeled and finely sliced
small knob of butter
1 tsp brown sugar or **honey**
8 anchovies
15–20 black olives

Preheat the oven to 180°C/Gas 4. Bring the stock to the boil in a large saucepan. Turn down the heat and slowly add the polenta, whisking constantly to avoid it becoming lumpy. Add the Parmesan and butter as you continue to whisk. Cook the polenta, stirring regularly, until it is very thick and comes away from the sides of the pan easily; this will take about 10 minutes.

Rub the bottom of a 23cm flan dish with olive oil, pour in the polenta and bake it for 30 minutes while you prepare the topping.

In a large frying pan, soften the onions in the olive oil and butter with the sugar over a very low heat. This always takes longer than you think – around 20 minutes – add a little bit of water if they get too dry.

When the onions are soft, spread them over the polenta and top with the anchovies and olives. Eat immediately or, if preparing ahead, warm in the oven just before serving.

dahl

MARIA PEREIRA, FROM GOA, INTRODUCED MY YOUNG TASTE BUDS TO THE
AROMATIC FLAVOURS OF INDIAN COOKING AND SHOWED ME HOW TO MAKE THIS
RECIPE. DAHL JUST MEANS 'LENTILS', SO IT'S ONE OF DOZENS OF RECIPES USING
THIS STAPLE. IF YOU LIKE DAHL HOT AS WELL AS SPICY, ADD A SHAKE OF CHILLI
POWDER TO TASTE WITH THE OTHER SPICES.

1 mugful of orange split
  lentils
1 large **onion**, *peeled and*
  chopped
5 **garlic** *cloves*
1 tsp olive oil
1 tsp ground coriander
1 tsp ground cumin
1 tsp ground **turmeric**
3 mugfuls of water
400g canned chopped
  tomatoes

Wash the lentils well in a sieve and check for any
grit lurking amongst them. In a large saucepan,
soften the onion and garlic in the olive oil with the
spices over a low heat. Don't allow the onion to
brown – if necessary, add a little water.

Add the lentils, water and tomatoes and bring
to the boil. Lower the heat and leave it all to
simmer for about an hour, stirring regularly to
make sure the bottom is not sticking. If the dahl
starts to become too thick, add a little more water.

Eat with brown basmati rice and steamed
broccoli or spinach.

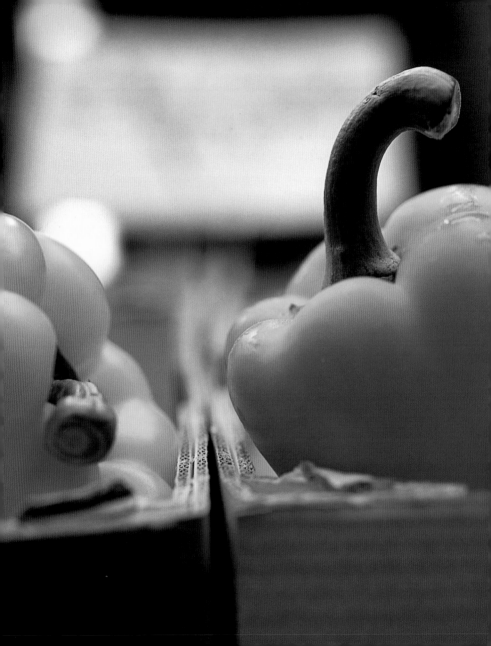

sweet pepper

The sweet pepper is a very versatile vegetable that can be eaten raw, in casseroles, roasted, stuffed and stir-fried. Their spicy cousins, chillies, have similar health benefits if you can stand the heat. Capsaicin, the substance in peppers that determines their hotness, has antibacterial and anti-inflammatory powers, and is a natural stimulant. In force, it is great for clearing the sinuses. Even in sweet peppers, the stimulation from capsaicin boosts the circulation and digestion. Peppers are also loaded with the powerful immune-boosting vitamins A and C, so they are good for fighting off infections or keeping them at bay in the first place. These vitamins are also needed for healthy skin and lungs, and cancer protection, although much of the vitamin C in peppers is lost when they are cooked. Despite all their goodness, as a member of the nightshade family, sweet peppers may exacerbate symptoms in those with arthritis and they can irritate the gut if there is a sensitivity problem.

seared tuna & peppers

QUICK, FRESH, SIMPLE, DELICIOUS ... AND GOOD FOR YOU.

*4 fresh **tuna** steaks*
*2 spring **onions**, trimmed*
*   and very finely sliced*
*1 tbsp **lemon** juice*
*10–12 **basil** leaves, chopped*
freshly ground black pepper
*1 red **pepper***
*1 yellow **pepper***
a little olive oil
***lemon** wedges, to serve*

Put the tuna steaks in a dish or bowl with the spring onions, lemon juice, chopped basil and some black pepper.

Halve the sweet peppers and remove the core and seeds, then slice lengthways. Heat a griddle pan and add a little olive oil. Add the peppers and cook, turning them regularly, for about 8 minutes.

Then move the peppers to one side and add the tuna to the griddle. Sprinkle with the marinade and sear it to your taste – a minute or so on each side, or longer if you want it cooked through.

Serve with lemon wedges, Tangy citrus cous cous (page 246) and a Wonderfoods green salad (page 111).

roasted red pepper purée

THIS SAUCE CAN BE EATEN WITH GRILLED OR SEARED FISH, CHICKEN OR LEAN MEAT. IT CAN EVEN BE TURNED INTO A SOUP, BY DOUBLING THE QUANTITIES AND ADDING SOME STOCK.

8 red **peppers**
4 **garlic** cloves (unpeeled)
1 **onion**, cut into eighths
    (unpeeled)
splash of olive oil
2 tsp ground coriander
few **thyme** sprigs
juice of ½ **lemon**

Preheat the oven to 180°C/Gas 4. Toss the whole peppers, garlic and onion in a roasting pan with a splash of olive oil, the ground coriander and thyme. Roast for about 30 minutes until the peppers are soft, then put them in a plastic bag, seal and leave to 'sweat' for about 5 minutes. Meanwhile, peel the onion and garlic cloves. Discard the thyme.

Take out the peppers and remove their stalks, seeds and skin (easiest done under running water). Put them in a blender with the garlic, onion and lemon juice and whiz to a purée.

NOTE If you're going to make a soup, tip the red pepper purée into a pan and add 400–500ml vegetable stock to thin it down to the required consistency. Heat it through gently to serve.

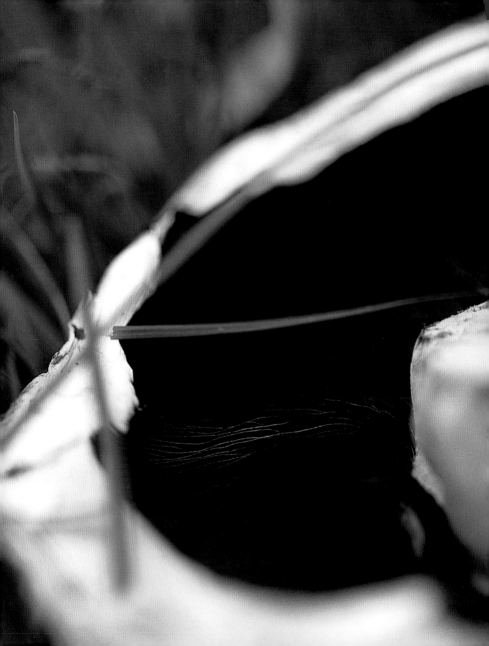

mushrooms

Scientists in Europe and America are only just tapping into the wonders of certain mushrooms that have been used medicinally in Japan and China for millennia. They have isolated polysaccharides such as lentinan in shiitake, maitake and reishi mushrooms, and shown them to power up the immune system dramatically. Not only are they strongly antibacterial and antiviral, but they have even been investigated for their potential in preventing and treating certain diseases, such as rheumatoid arthritis, cancer and HIV. In addition to these immune-boosting powerful compounds, such mushrooms are also a good source of some B vitamins, iron and zinc, which is needed for making energy and fighting off infections. Shiitake contain another active component, eritadenine, which has been shown to lower cholesterol. Even if you can't get these mushrooms fresh, dried ones store well and are a tasty addition to soups, casseroles, risottos, stir-fries, sauces and even roasts. That way you still benefit from nature's synergy of all the compounds, some probably unknown.

hot & sour mushroom broth

THIS RECIPE IS BASED ON THE THAI SOUP *TOM YUM*. IT TAKES NO TIME TO MAKE, DESPITE THE LENGTHY INGREDIENTS LIST. IF YOU'RE USING DRIED SHIITAKE, YOU'LL NEED TO MAKE SURE THE SOUP SIMMERS FOR LONG ENOUGH TO REHYDRATE THEM WELL. TO MAKE IT MORE FILLING, ADD A GOOD HANDFUL OF RICE NOODLES.

*5 tbsp miso (**soya** paste)*
1.5 litres boiling water
*200g shiitake **mushrooms***
2 small red, fresh chillies,
*   deseeded and sliced*
1 lemongrass stalk, sliced
2.5cm piece fresh root
*   **ginger**, peeled and*
*   grated*
2.5cm piece fresh galangal,
*   peeled and sliced*
*   (optional)*
3 dried kaffir lime leaves
*4 spring **onions**, trimmed*
*   and sliced*
1 tbsp Thai fish sauce
1 tbsp tamari or soy sauce
*1 tbsp **lime** juice*
2 tsp brown sugar or
*   alternative equivalent*
*   (see page 10)*
*200g **spinach** leaves,*
*   washed and roughly torn*
coriander leaves, torn,
*   to garnish*

In a large pan, mix the miso paste with a little of the boiling water, then stir in the remaining water. Add the rest of the ingredients, except the spinach and coriander, and bring to the boil. Immediately turn the heat down and simmer gently for about 10 minutes. Add the spinach at the last minute.

Serve the broth scattered with freshly torn coriander. It tastes even better the next day.

mushroom baked chicken

THIS IS PRETTY MUCH THE ROAST CHICKEN STAPLE IN OUR HOUSE, USUALLY WITH A WHOLE CHICKEN COOKED IN AN OLD TERRACOTTA POT.

1 **onion**, peeled and sliced
2 tbsp dried **seaweed**
12 shiitake **mushrooms**, sliced
1cm piece fresh root **ginger**, peeled and grated
4 **chicken** breasts or 8 thighs
2 tbsp tamari or soy sauce
½ **lemon**
freshly ground black pepper

Preheat the oven to 190°C/Gas 5. Randomly scatter the onion in the bottom of a large baking dish with the crumbled, dried seaweed, the mushrooms and the ginger and put the chicken pieces on top. Drizzle the tamari and squeeze the lemon over the chicken, then put the spent lemon half in the dish. Season it all with pepper.

Pour in enough water to cover the mushrooms and seaweed. Bake for 30–40 minutes or until the chicken pieces are cooked through.

Eat with Scented savoury rice (page 67) and steamed or stir-fried green veg.

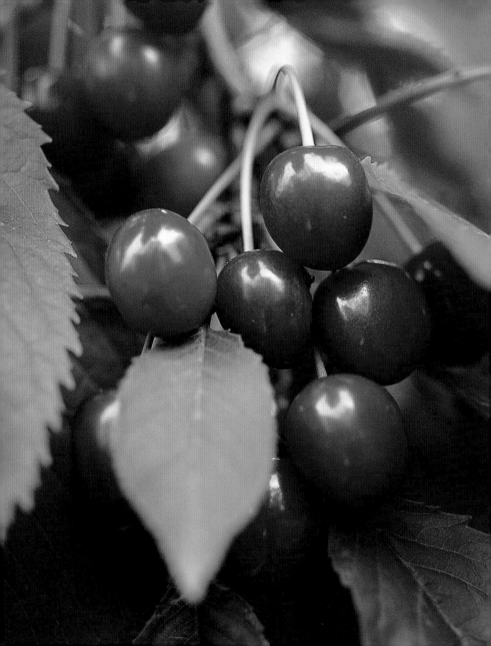

cherries

Cherries conjure up images of summer idyll, luxury and the memory of dangling double-stalked fruit over my ears as a child. It so happens that they are wonderfully good for you too. As their deep, rich red colour suggests, they are packed with powerful antioxidant compounds that support the body's immune system, fight arthritis and can even help to protect against cancer and heart disease. Cherries are also rich in flavonoids called anthocyanins and quercetin, which is notably strongly anti-inflammatory. Quercetin helps relieve painful inflammation of the joints, gout and allergic reactions involving histamine; it's been shown to help reduce the formation of cataracts, too. The key antioxidants in cherries work alongside vitamin C to help ward off viruses (including the common cold) and to strengthen collagen, our cellular support structure that in effect holds our skin, blood vessels, indeed our entire bodies together. Cherries are also a good source of several vitamins, including carotene, and minerals such as iron.

cherry chicken

YOU CAN EITHER REMOVE THE STONES FROM THE CHERRIES OR SAVE THE EFFORT
AND LEAVE THEM IN — JUST REMEMBER TO WARN EVERYONE BEFORE EATING!
IF FRESH CHERRIES ARE OUT OF SEASON, OPT FOR UNSWEETENED FROZEN ONES
INSTEAD. FOR AN ALCOHOL-FREE VERSION, USE WATER RATHER THAN WINE.

½ **onion**, peeled and sliced
1 tsp olive oil
8 star anise
4 **chicken** breasts with skin
(or thighs or drumsticks)
2 tbsp tamari or soy sauce
1 tbsp **honey**
100ml freshly squeezed
orange juice
2 tbsp balsamic vinegar
100ml red wine
300g **cherries**

Preheat the oven to 180°C/Gas 4. In a flameproof
casserole, soften the onion in the olive oil together
with the star anise. Add the chicken and cook for
2–3 minutes on each side until lightly coloured.
Stir in the tamari, honey, orange juice, balsamic
vinegar and wine. Bring to the boil, lower the heat
and simmer for 4–5 minutes.

Tip in the cherries and stir to mix. Cover and
cook in the oven for 20 minutes, then squish the
cherries into the sauce to make it darker and
more flavourful. Bake, uncovered, for a further
20–25 minutes or until the chicken is tender. Serve
with brown rice and steamed green veg.

chocolatey cherries

THESE MAKE A TEMPTING LIGHT DESSERT, OR YOU CAN SERVE THEM WITH MINT TEA (OR COFFEE) AFTER DINNER. YOU NEED RIPE CHERRIES AND GOOD QUALITY CHOCOLATE THAT'S AT LEAST 70% COCOA SOLIDS. USE HALF CHERRIES AND HALF STRAWBERRIES IF YOU LIKE.

500g **cherries**, with stalks
200g dark **chocolate**

Rinse and dry the cherries. Line a baking tray with greaseproof paper. Break up the chocolate into a heatproof bowl and rest the bowl on top of a pan of gently simmering water, making sure the base of the bowl doesn't touch the water. Leave until the chocolate is melted, then stir until smooth.

Holding it by the stalk, dip each cherry into the melted chocolate to coat and then place on the lined baking tray. Leave until the chocolate has set.

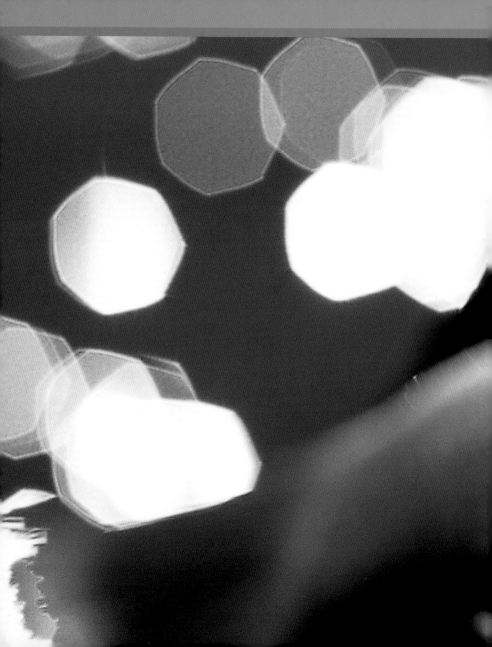

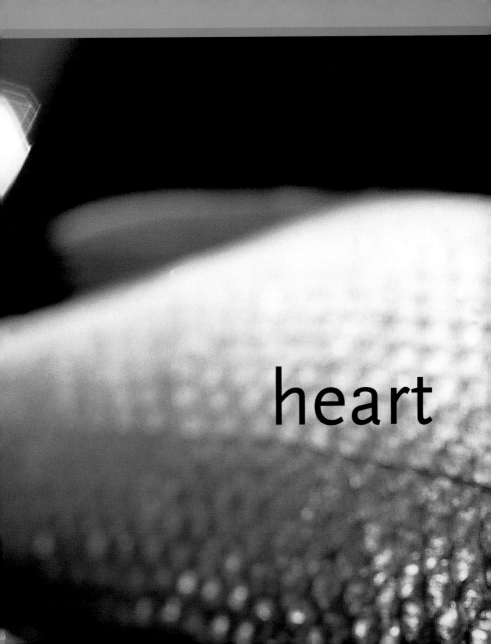

heart

The wonderfoods in this section are just a few of those that play a particularly important part in keeping all the various forms of cardiovascular disease (CVD) at bay. CVD is rife in the so-called 'developed' countries where we have acquired diets and lifestyles that leave us riddled with conditions that slowly kill us. Diseases of the heart and blood vessels in the form of high blood pressure, thickening of the arteries, deposits in the arteries, inflammation in artery walls, blood clots and high cholesterol build up silently. These all clog up the arteries that supply the brain, heart and other vital organs, resulting in heart attacks and strokes. All authorities on heart disease recognise that we do really have significant control over the degree to which any of these progress.

As you will see from the individual wonderfood entries, some help regulate blood pressure by contributing to the mineral balance in the body, acting as a diuretic or relaxing blood vessels. Others help reduce the likelihood of blood clotting unnecessarily, which contributes to strokes and heart attacks. The build up of cholesterol in the lining of blood vessels, particularly when it is oxidised and therefore damaged (see age introduction, page 170), is recognised as a major contributing factor to heart disease. As you will discover, many of these heart wonderfoods help to reduce the build-up of 'harmful' cholesterol.

It is increasingly acknowledged that inflammation of the blood vessels underlies much CVD, and the wonderfoods here and others throughout the book help keep this down. Obviously, we need our blood to clot in certain situations such as when we cut or graze ourselves. However, over-stickiness of the blood makes it more liable to form clots inside the body and these can be dangerous as they create blockages. This is particularly hazardous if this occurs in the brain (such as in a stroke) or in the blood supply to the heart.

The insidious nature of CVD is such that it creeps up on us and we only usually find out about it when it is established, so prevention is the key, as it is with most illnesses. That's not to say it's too late to make a difference if you have already been diagnosed with, say, high blood pressure or high cholesterol. Eating the wonderfoods here and throughout the book can play a key role as it's indisputable that we can minimise our risk of succumbing to heart disease by eating healthily as well as exercising regularly, not smoking, not drinking excessive amounts of alcohol and maintaining our ideal weight.

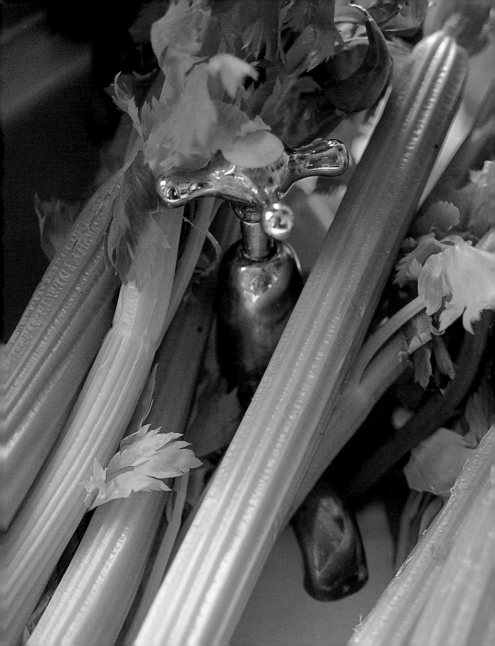

celery

Celery is as at home in a herbalist's apothecary as it is in the kitchen. Herbally, it is most widely used for helping to lower blood pressure on two fronts. One is because of its powerful diuretic action. The other is down to substances called phthalides, which help dilate blood vessels and that are, in general, relaxing. Celery is especially useful for people who suffer from water retention, because apart from its diuretic action, its potassium-sodium balance helps to regulate the body's fluids. Celery provides a decent amount of vitamin C, and valuable chemicals called coumarins, which have anti-cancer properties. Given that salt is linked to increasing blood pressure, it may seem somewhat contradictory that celery has a high organic sodium content that gives it a salty flavour and makes it useful for dislodging calcified build-ups in the joints. Strongly alkaline, celery is detoxifying and calming on the digestive system, and for many years it has been traditionally used to treat rheumatic and arthritic conditions, as well as gout.

crispy bean salad

THIS IS A STAPLE LUNCH IN OUR HOUSE — IT'S EASY TO MAKE AND VERY PORTABLE TOO. YOU COULD VARY THE FLAVOUR BY USING DIFFERENT OILS OR HERBS, SUCH AS SESAME OIL AND CORIANDER WITH A DASH OF TABASCO.

2 x 400g can **beans** (pinto, borlotti or mixed), drained and rinsed

2 medium **tomatoes**, roughly chopped

4 spring **onions**, trimmed and sliced

4 **celery** sticks, finely sliced

pinch of sea salt

2 tbsp olive oil

1 tbsp **lemon** juice

2 tbsp finely chopped **parsley**

In a large bowl, mix the beans together with all the other ingredients and eat it — just like that!

chicken & rocket salad

THIS MAKES A GOOD WEEKEND SUMMER LUNCH. YOU CAN COOK THE CHICKEN
BREASTS IN ADVANCE TO PILE ON TOP OF THE SALAD ANY TIME.

4 skinless boneless **chicken**
breasts
2 tsp pesto
4 handfuls of rocket leaves
4 **celery** *sticks, finely sliced*
8 cherry **tomatoes***, halved*
1 **avocado***, peeled, stoned*
and cubed
FOR THE VINAIGRETTE
2 tbsp balsamic vinegar
1 heaped tsp Dijon mustard
6 tbsp olive oil
freshly ground black pepper

Preheat the oven to 200°C/Gas 6. Spread the
chicken breasts all over with the pesto and lay
them in an ovenproof dish. Add enough water to
just cover the bottom of the dish. Bake for about
25 minutes until the chicken is cooked through:
test with a skewer – the juices should run clear.

Meanwhile, assemble the salad ingredients. To
make the vinaigrette, put the balsamic vinegar and
mustard in a screw-topped jar and shake well,
then add the olive oil and pepper and shake again.

When the chicken is cooked, pile the salad
ingredients on to four plates and drizzle about
1 tbsp vinaigrette over each portion. Slice the
chicken breasts and arrange on top of the salad.
Serve at once.

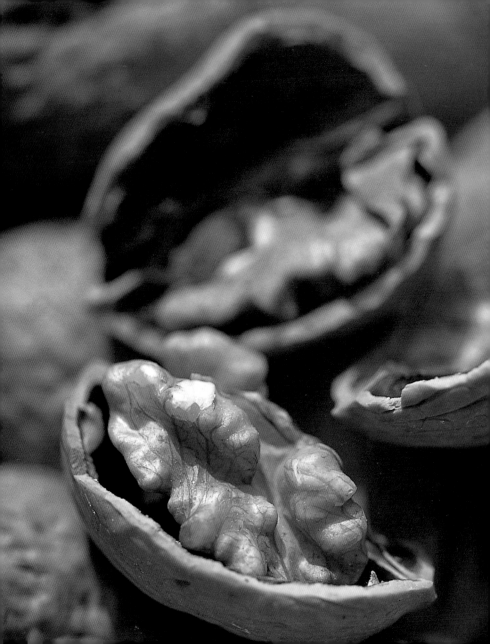

walnuts

Apparently walnuts were eaten by Jupiter and other gods, who would have gained from more than just their taste. These nuts are loaded with essential fatty acids, EFAs, particularly the omega 6s, but also omega 3s and monounsaturates (like olive oil). Omega 3s have a host of benefits for the cardiovascular system. They lower LDL cholesterol (the 'bad' type) improving its ratio to HDL (the 'good' type), lower lipoprotein A (another 'baddie'), make blood less likely to clot and increase the elasticity of arteries. Arginine, an amino acid in walnuts, also helps blood vessels relax, reducing the chance of high blood pressure. Antioxidant chemicals such as ellagic acid protect cholesterol from oxidative damage, as well as conferring anti-cancer properties. EFAs also make for better nerve transmission (needed for good memory and moods), keep skin smooth and calm inflammation in conditions such as asthma, arthritis, eczema and psoriasis. On top of all this, walnuts contain the minerals copper, manganese, iron and zinc, as well as fibre and B vitamins.

pear & walnut sweet polenta

THIS IS AN UNUSUAL, VERY EASY 'FLAN', WHICH CAN BE EATEN AS A DESSERT OR
EVEN AT TEATIME.

100ml **apple** juice
400ml water
2 tbsp **honey** or maple
    syrup
3 ripe but firm **pears**, cored
    and sliced
150g 'instant' polenta or
    cornmeal
1 tsp butter
a little olive oil, to brush
about 20 **walnuts**, broken
    up
TO SERVE
150g natural **yoghurt**
½ tsp vanilla extract, or
    to taste

Preheat the oven to 180°C/Gas 4. Pour the apple
juice and water into a large saucepan, add the
honey and bring to the boil. Turn down the heat
and add the pear slices. Simmer for 6–7 minutes,
then remove the pears with a slotted spoon and
set aside.

Slowly add the polenta to the liquid in the pan,
whisking constantly to avoid it getting lumpy. Add
the butter as you whisk. Continue to cook the
polenta, stirring regularly, until it is very thick and
comes away from the sides of the pan easily,
about 10 minutes.

Rub the bottom of a 23cm flan dish with olive
oil, pour in the polenta and bake for 30 minutes.
Lay the pear slices on the polenta, scatter the
walnuts over the top and return to the oven for
15 minutes. Meanwhile, flavour the yoghurt with a
few drops of vanilla extract to taste.

Cut the 'flan' into slices and eat warm with the
vanilla-flavoured yoghurt or soured cream.

savoury walnut pâté

THIS CAN BE EATEN ON CRACKERS OR TOAST, OR EVEN WITH CRUDITÉS AS A DIP.

150g **walnuts**
handful of **parsley**, plus
   sprigs to garnish
150g feta cheese, crumbled
120ml water
1 small **garlic** clove, peeled
1 tsp ground coriander
few shakes of cayenne
   pepper
a little olive oil

Put the walnuts and parsley in a blender and pulse until the nuts are ground. Then add the feta, water, garlic, coriander and cayenne and whiz briefly until smooth.

Spoon into a serving dish, drizzle with a little olive oil and top with a few parsley sprigs.

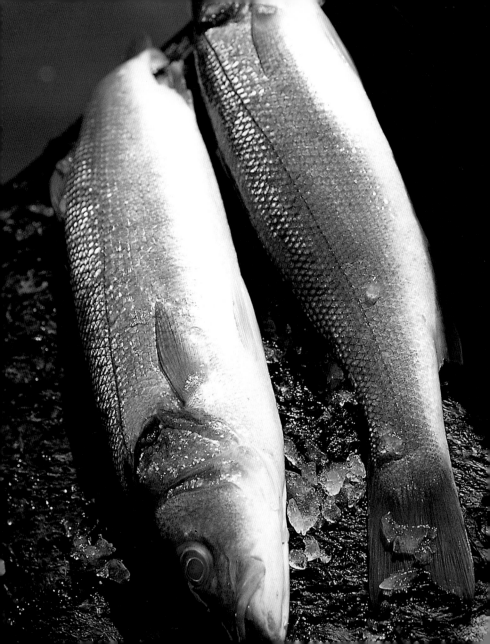

fish

Fish are not only heart food, but a total wonderfood. All are an excellent source of protein and oily fish — fresh tuna, salmon, sardines, herring, mackerel, trout — are rich sources of the omega 3 essential fatty acids (EFAs), DHA (docosahexaenoic acid) and EPA (eicosapentaenoic acid). These fats are renowned for reducing heart attacks and factors that contribute to cardiovascular disease, such as blood clotting and high blood pressure. EFAS are integrated into cell membranes, so not only do they make your skin smooth, they also help the function of every single cell. DHA is especially important in the brain and nervous system, helping to improve learning, to combat age-related memory decline, and to enhance mood. EFAs also have powerful anti-inflammatory properties, making them useful in conditions such as arthritis, asthma and eczema. Fish is a source of sulphur, a valuable mineral for detoxification. It also contains choline, a B vitamin family member, needed for healthy cell membranes and for the formation of the body's own memory messenger, the neurotransmitter, acetylcholine.

fish kebabs

YOU CAN VARY THESE KEBABS BY CHOOSING DIFFERENT FISH OR PERHAPS
CHICKEN OR LAMB, AND OTHER VEGETABLES SUCH AS PAR-BOILED CHUNKS OF
CORN-ON-THE-COB OR ROASTED SWEET POTATOES.

200g **monkfish** fillet, cubed
200g **salmon** fillet, cubed
4 large scallops, shelled and
    cleaned
4 large raw prawns, shelled
    but with tails left on
1 red **pepper**, deseeded and
    cut into squares
1 yellow **pepper**, deseeded
    and cut into squares
2 courgettes, sliced into 1cm
    chunks
FOR THE MARINADE
juice of 3 **limes**
freshly ground black pepper
3 tbsp olive oil
$^1/_2$ tsp ground **turmeric**
$^1/_2$ tsp ground cumin
1 tsp Tabasco sauce

In a large dish, mix all the marinade ingredients
together. Add the cubed fish, scallops and prawns,
turning to coat them well. Leave to stand for about
20 minutes.

Preheat the grill. Remove the fish and shellfish
from the dish, reserving the marinade. Thread
them on to four skewers, alternating with the
vegetables. Grill the kebabs for about 3 minutes
on each side until the fish is cooked, basting them
with the marinade as you turn them.

Serve on brown rice (cooked in fish stock
rather than water for extra flavour if you like) and
a Wonderfoods green salad (page 111).

NOTE If you use wooden rather than metal
skewers, you will need to soak them in advance
to prevent them from scorching under the grill.

nellie fish

THIS WAY OF COOKING FISH IS A STAPLE AT THE HOME OF MY FRIENDS, NELLIE
AND MICHAEL. IT'S MY FAVOURITE WAY OF COOKING HALIBUT, THOUGH I OFTEN
USE HADDOCK FOR A CHEAPER OPTION.

16–20 cherry **tomatoes**
2 tbsp olive oil
8 **garlic** cloves (unpeeled)
2 red or green chillies
1 tbsp tamari or soy sauce
4 fillets of any **fish** you like,
    each about 175g

Preheat the oven to 200°C/Gas 6. Put the cherry
tomatoes, olive oil, garlic cloves, whole chillies
and tamari in a large ovenproof dish, toss well
and bake the lot for about 20 minutes until the
tomatoes are slightly wrinkled.

Add the fish fillets, swishing them around in
the dish and turning to coat them on both sides
with the mixture. Bake for 15–20 minutes until the
fish is cooked, depending on the size of the fillets.
Discard the chillies.

Eat with a Wonderfoods green salad (page 111)
and boiled buckwheat, squeezing out the garlic on
to the fish and tomatoes as you eat them.

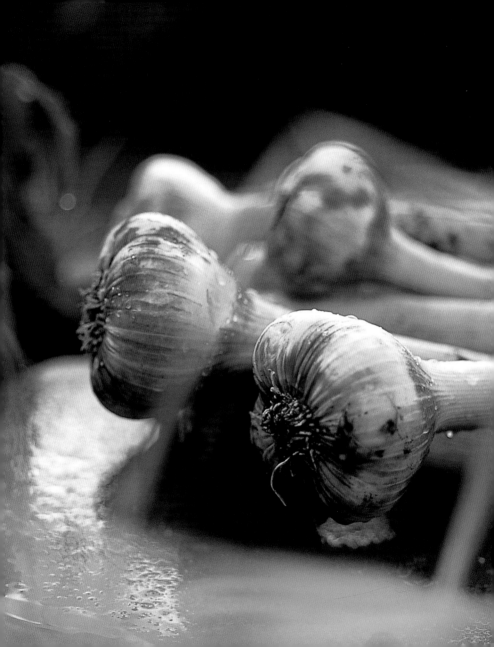

garlic

Ancient records in Asia show that garlic has been valued for thousands of years as a potent medicine with powers as far reaching as an aphrodisiac, a purifier, healer and strength-builder. Heart-wise, garlic is a megastar. It helps prevent hardening of arteries, reduces LDL cholesterol and blood fats while increasing HDL, deters the clumping of blood cells, lowers blood pressure and helps prevent harmful oxidative damage to cholesterol. Many of its benefits derive from sulphur compounds, such as allicin, that are also powerful detoxifiers for the liver and lymph system as well as anti-inflammatories. Garlic is also a powerful antibiotic, helping clear bacterial, fungal, worm and amoebic infections in the digestive tract. This property, plus its immune-boosting role and decongestant effect, enables garlic to ward off viral and other infections throughout the body, including coughs and colds. It also helps to protect against cancer. To get the most, healthwise, from garlic, it's best eaten raw – in salads or mixed into dishes after they have been cooked.

som tam

THIS IS A MILD VERSION OF ONE OF MY FAVOURITE DISHES EVER. TRADITIONALLY FROM NORTH-EAST THAILAND, IT'S MADE TO ORDER WITH A PESTLE AND MORTAR AT STREET STALLS AND SERVED WITH STICKY RICE AND GRILLED CHICKEN. VISIT YOUR LOCAL ASIAN GROCERS TO GET THE INGREDIENTS. IF YOU CAN'T FIND GREEN PAPAYA, USE HALF A WHITE CABBAGE INSTEAD.

2 **garlic** cloves
1 bird's eye chilli
2 tsp coconut palm sugar
    (jaggery from Indian
    grocers)
2 tbsp roasted peanuts (not
    salted)
10 green beans, sliced
4 cherry **tomatoes**
½ green **papaya**, peeled,
    deseeded and finely
    shredded
juice of 2 **limes**
2 tsp tamarind concentrate,
    diluted with 2 tsp water
1 tbsp Thai fish sauce

Using a pestle and mortar, crush the garlic, chilli, palm sugar and peanuts together. Add the beans and tomatoes, pounding all the time. Bit by bit, add the shredded papaya, still pounding.

Slowly add the lime juice, then the tamarind juice and fish sauce, continuing to pound. Taste and add a little more lime and tamarind if you want a sharper flavour. Eat it straight away, with grilled chicken and rice.

roasted garlic & tomato soup

THIS IS A VERY DENSE, WARMING SOUP, ALTHOUGH YOU COULD THIN IT DOWN
WITH EXTRA STOCK OR WATER IF YOU WANTED SOMETHING LIGHTER.

2 **garlic** bulbs, broken into
    cloves (unpeeled)
10 medium-large **tomatoes**
splash of olive oil
500ml vegetable or chicken
    stock
10–12 **basil** leaves
2 tbsp **lemon** juice
1/2 tsp cayenne pepper

Preheat the oven to 200°C/Gas 6. Toss the garlic cloves and tomatoes in a splash of olive oil in an ovenproof dish. Roast them for 40 minutes.

Peel away the skins from the roasted garlic cloves and tomatoes, then put them in a large saucepan with the stock, basil leaves, lemon juice and cayenne. Bring to the boil, then whiz it all up using a hand-held stick blender.

Serve the soup hot, with chunks of rye bread.

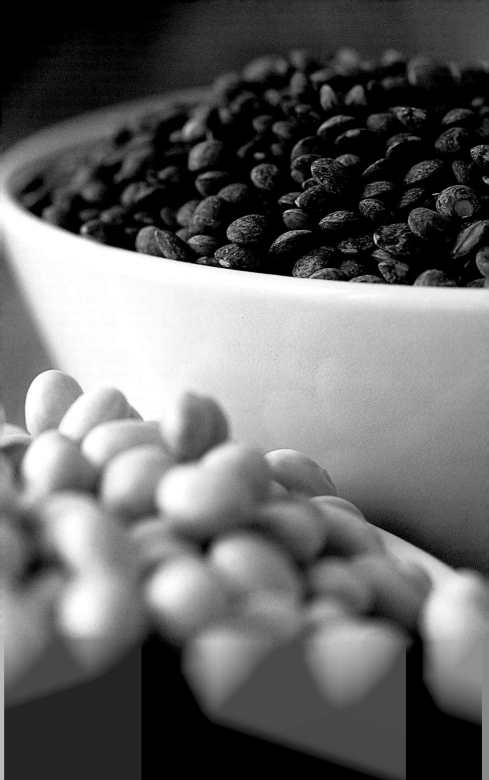

lentils & beans

Not the easiest of foods to digest, beans and lentils have a valid reputation for inducing wind, but they have hidden talents. Scientists have shown that eating such high fibre foods dramatically lowers the risk of heart disease. One reason is that fibre binds with cholesterol in the gut and ferries it out of the body. Plenty of fibre also means that blood sugar levels don't rise rapidly after eating, keeping insulin from shooting up – especially useful for people with diabetes or other blood sugar problems. Rising insulin levels stimulate the production of cholesterol and people with diabetes have a greater risk of cardiovascular disease. Beans contain folic acid, which helps lower the chemical homocysteine, high levels of which are linked to heart disease, Alzheimer's and depression. All in all, beans and lentils are a low fat, low calorie, dense source of fibre, protein, vitamins and minerals. To reduce their wind potential, soak lentils and beans well before cooking and then use fresh water to boil, or cook them with some kombu seaweed and ginger, or sprout them (see page 110).

warm puy lentil salad

YOU CAN EAT THIS SALAD WARM OR COLD. THE COLD-PRESSED SUNFLOWER OIL
ADDS A NUTTY TOUCH — IF YOU CAN'T GET HOLD OF IT, DOUBLE THE AMOUNT OF
OLIVE OIL RATHER THAN USE REGULAR SUPERMARKET SUNFLOWER OIL.

1½ mugfuls of Puy **lentils**
3 medium **tomatoes**
3 spring **onions**, trimmed
   and finely sliced
10–12 **basil** leaves, roughly
   torn
1 tbsp olive oil
1 tbsp cold-pressed
   sunflower oil
2 tsp balsamic vinegar
freshly ground black pepper
pinch of salt

Wash the lentils and put them in a large saucepan.
Add water to cover generously and bring to the
boil. Lower the heat and leave to simmer for about
30 minutes until the lentils are tender.

While they are cooking, drop the tomatoes into
the pan for a minute to loosen the skins, then
remove with a slotted spoon and peel away the
skins. Roughly chop the tomato flesh.

Drain the lentils well and toss them with the
tomatoes and all the other ingredients. Serve with
a Wonderfoods green salad (page 111).

fruity baked beans

30.6.07

THIS IS INSPIRED BY A RECIPE IN THE VEGETARIAN MOOSEWOOD COOKBOOK BY
MOLLIE KATZEN. I SOMETIMES ADD LEAN, CHUNKY BACON TO MAKE IT EVEN
HEARTIER ON A WINTER'S NIGHT. IDEALLY, YOU COOK DRIED BEANS FIRST BUT,
LET'S FACE IT, NOT MANY OF US GET ROUND TO THAT.

3 **onions**, peeled and sliced
1 tbsp olive oil
2 tsp ground coriander
1 tsp smoked paprika
1 tsp cayenne pepper
2 large cooking **apples**,
    peeled, cored and cut
    into 1cm chunks
4 medium **tomatoes**,
    skinned and chopped
8 **garlic** cloves, peeled and
    crushed
6 tbsp cider vinegar
3 tbsp molasses or **honey**
2 star anise
3 x 420g cans of haricot or
    borlotti **beans**, drained

Preheat the oven to 180°C/Gas 4. In a large
saucepan, soften the onions in the olive oil with
the ground coriander, paprika and cayenne for
about 10 minutes. Add the apples, tomatoes,
garlic, vinegar, molasses and star anise. Stir and
cook for 4–5 minutes before adding the beans.

Transfer the lot to a casserole dish, cover and
cook in the oven for an hour.

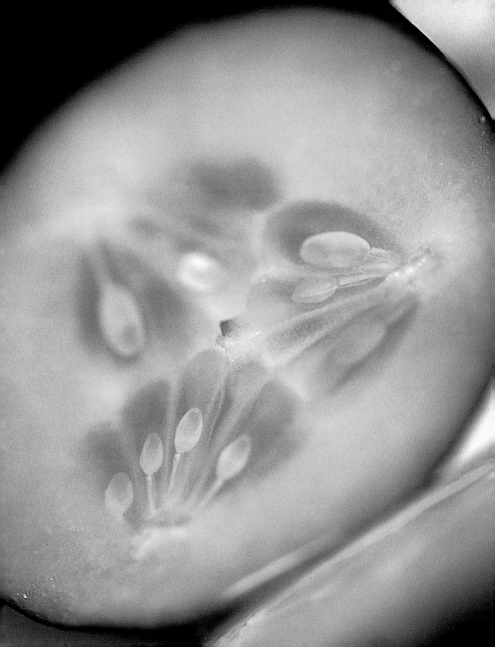

cucumber

This water-laden member of the gourd family (related to courgettes, pumpkin and watermelon) has been popular since ancient times, not just as a food but also for its skin-healing properties. Its high water and balanced mineral content makes cucumber one of the best-known diuretics – it helps the body eliminate water, which in turn keeps blood pressure down. This 'flushing' of water through the kidneys also means that cucumber is a good detoxifier, helping the body eliminate waste products. A high water intake also helps keep the bowels moving well. The advice to drink however many litres of water a day doesn't often take into account the water in foods; if you eat plenty of fruits and vegetables like cucumbers, you don't need to drink quite so much water. Cucumbers are rich in silica, a mineral needed for healthy skin, bone and all connective tissues in the body; also the somewhat obscure mineral molybdenum, which is needed for detoxification. Cucumbers also provide a range of other nutrients such as vitamin C, potassium, magnesium and fibre.

cucumber fettuccine salad

THIS SALAD GOES WELL WITH CARROT FELAFEL (PAGE 183) AND IS A GOOD
ACCOMPANIMENT TO JERUSALEM CHICKEN (PAGE 34). IT DOESN'T CONTAIN
FETTUCCINE, BUT TAKES ITS NAME FROM THE FINE-CUT CUCUMBER RIBBONS.

1 long cucumber
1 tbsp chopped mint
2 tbsp chopped parsley
2 tbsp lemon juice
2 tbsp olive oil
200g natural cottage cheese
freshly ground black pepper
pinch of sea salt

Using a swivel potato peeler, pare the cucumber into long, fine ribbons, dropping them on to a clean tea towel. Pat them to remove some of the liquid, discard the outer skin pieces, then tip into a large bowl. Add all the other ingredients, toss lightly to mix, then serve.

spicy tuna & cucumber salad

A FAIL-SAFE RECIPE — YOU COULD USE ANY FISH YOU FANCY REALLY.

4 fresh **tuna** steaks, each
   about 150g
FOR THE MARINADE
1 tbsp Tabasco sauce
1 tbsp **lemon** juice
1 tbsp olive oil
2 **garlic** cloves, peeled and
   crushed
FOR THE SALAD
1 long **cucumber**, cut into
   5mm slices
1 red **pepper**, cored,
   deseeded and finely
   sliced
2 tbsp **lemon** juice
2 tbsp olive oil
1 tbsp chopped coriander
2 tsp tamari or soy sauce

Combine the marinade ingredients in a shallow dish, add the tuna steaks and turn to coat. Leave the fish to marinate for about 30 minutes.

Meanwhile, make the salad. Toss all the ingredients together in a bowl and then divide between four plates.

Preheat a griddle pan. Sear the tuna steaks for about 2 minutes on each side or until cooked to your liking. Lay the tuna steaks on top of the salad and serve immediately.

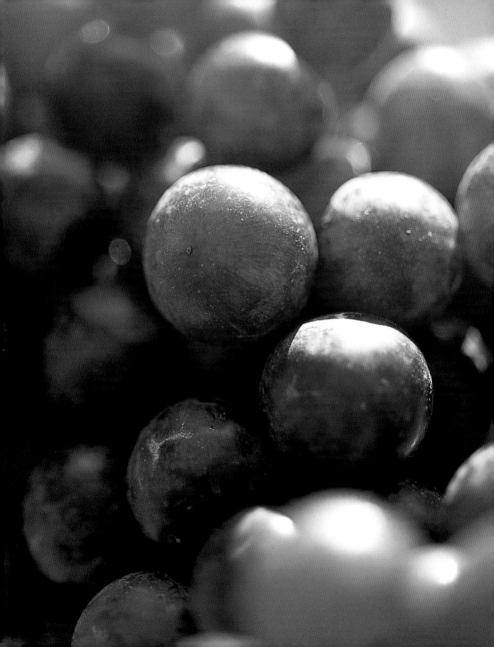

grapes

In ancient literature you'll find tales of grapes, their symbolism and their association with wine and hedonism, and now current scientific literature abounds on their remarkable health benefits. Grapes contain antioxidant flavonoid compounds that not only protect against heart disease, but also cancer and ageing. Saponins, pterostilbene, resveratrol and other substances contribute in many ways to cutting the risk of heart disease by reducing platelet clumping and blood clots, dropping blood pressure, lowering LDL cholesterol, inhibiting the oxidation of LDL, relaxing blood vessels, preventing the heart muscle from stiffening and reducing inflammation, which is increasingly recognised as a cause of cardiovascular problems. Resveratrol in particular is exciting scientists as a cancer-preventative agent. The water and fibre in grapes makes them useful against constipation and for detoxifying the gut and liver. Get the benefits from grapes themselves and grape juice (especially red), rather than wine as the alcohol and preservatives can trigger migraines and other problems.

scallop, grape & grapefruit salad

IF YOU CAN GET FRESH SCALLOPS, THIS IS A FINE, REFRESHING SALAD. OTHERWISE
YOU COULD SUBSTITUTE PRAWNS OR BITE-SIZED PIECES OF CHICKEN INSTEAD.

16–20 red **grapes**, washed
1 pink **grapefruit**
4 handfuls of **watercress**,
    washed
16 large scallops, shelled
    and cleaned
a little olive oil
FOR THE DRESSING
4 tbsp **grapefruit** juice
1 tbsp olive oil
1 tbsp sweet chilli sauce

Halve the grapes and remove the pips. Peel and
segment the grapefruit, discarding all membrane
and pith. Arrange the grapes, grapefruit and
watercress on four plates.

Shake the dressing ingredients together in a
screw-topped jar.

Preheat a griddle pan and oil it very lightly.
Sear the scallops in the hot pan for about 1 minute
each side and then lay them on top of the salad.
Drizzle a little dressing over each portion and eat
immediately.

frosted grapes

YOU COULDN'T GET MUCH SIMPLER THAN THIS!

handful of green **grapes**, washed
handful of red **grapes**, washed
few splashes of sweet wine, brandy or apple juice

Lay the grapes on a tray or in a large plastic container and put them in the freezer overnight. Get them out of the freezer and eat them straight away, drizzled with a little sweet wine, brandy or apple juice.

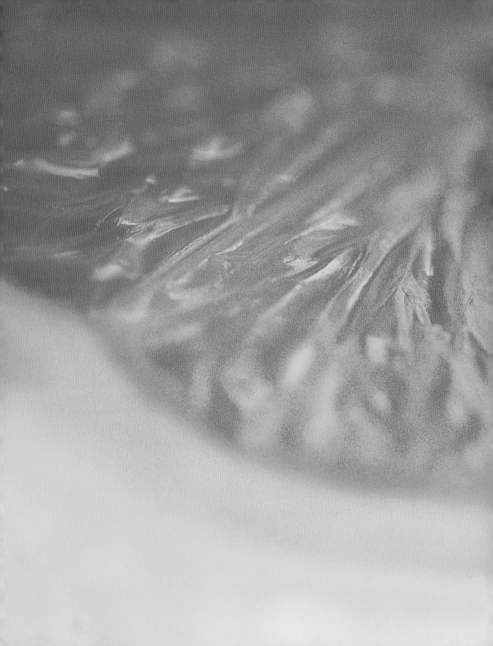

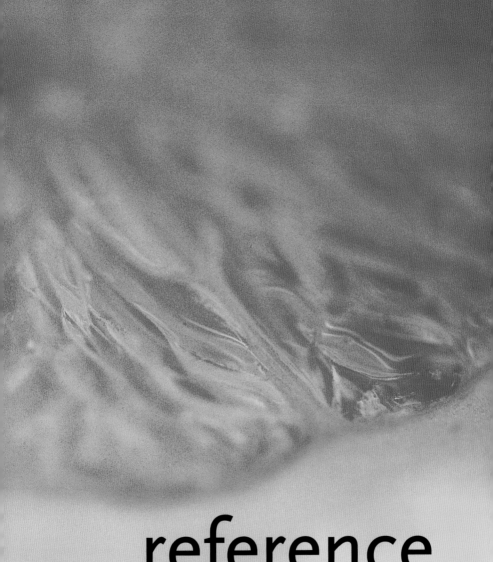

reference

wonderfoods week

YOU COULD EASILY GO THROUGH AN ENTIRE WEEK EATING MEALS MADE UP OF
WONDERFOODS. HERE'S JUST A SAMPLE IDEA OF HOW...

	Breakfast	Lighter Meal	Main Meal	Dessert/Teatime
Mon	Honeyed granola (page 38)	Papaya & prawn salad (page 54)	Lemongrass turkey skewers (page 210)	Apple custard tart (page 51)
Tues	Blackcurrant smoothie (page 238)	Artichoke heart pizzas (page 107)	Soba noodles & salmon (page 75)	Mango with coconut rice (page 31)
Wed	Scrambled eggs with watercress (page 203)	Marinated red onion & beetroot salad (page 90)	Jerusalem chicken (page 34)	Blackcurrant & apricot slice (page 239)
Thurs	Spiced apricots (page 174)	Frittata tricolore (page 150)	Mackerel with apple purée (page 50)	Blueberry cheesecake (page 178)
Fri	Mango incognito (page 179)	Kiwi & figs with Parma ham (page 190)	White bean mash (page 199)	Roasted pears with lime & ginger (page 79)
Sat	Fruity porridge (page 223)	Broccoli polenta flan (page 227)	Seed-crusted monkfish in Parma ham (page 147)	Orange almond torte (page 118)
Sun	Buckwheat crêpes (page 74)	Hot & sour mushroom broth (page 258)	Moroccan lamb (page 194)	Griddled papaya with lime honey (page 55)

wonderfoods contacts

FIND LOCAL FARM SHOPS AND ORGANIC DELIVERY SERVICES BY RECOMMENDATION OR BY SEARCHING THE WEB OR YOUR BOOKSHOP FOR AN ORGANIC DIRECTORY. OTHERWISE, JUST CHOOSE THE FRESHEST, BEST QUALITY PRODUCE THAT YOU CAN FIND AND AFFORD, IDEALLY LOCALLY PRODUCED AND ORGANIC.

Natalie Savona's nutrition work
For information, visit www.nataliesavona.com

National Farmers' Retail & Markets Association (FARMA)
A website of the organisation that governs and promotes farmers' markets throughout the UK.
www.farmersmarkets.net
Tel: 0845 230 2150

Henry Doubleday Research Organisation
The HRDA is dedicated to researching and promoting organic gardening, farming and food. Includes advice on organic gardening, information and its Heritage Seed Library.
www.hdra.org.uk
Tel: 024 7630 8202

The Soil Association
UK's leading organisation for the campaigning for and certification of organic food.
www.soilassociation.org
Tel: 0117 314 5000

Slow Food
International organisation aiming to preserve artisanal foods and regional traditions.
www.slowfood.com
Tel: 0800 917 1232

Brogdale Horticultural Trust
Home to the national fruit collection. Source of advice and stocks of a wide range of fruits that can grow in the UK including over 2000 varieties of apple.
www.brogdale.org
email: info@brogdale.org
Tel: 01795 535286

Nutrilink Ltd
Mail order supplier of useful products, including the sugar alternative xylitol (brand name Miracle Sweet).
Tel: 08704 054 002

OTHER READING
The Whole Foods Companion Dianne Onstad (Chelsea Green Publishing, Vermont, USA)
Herbal Deni Brown (Pavilion Books, London)
Cabbages & Kings Jonathan Roberts (HarperCollins, London)
The Kitchen Shrink Natalie Savona (Duncan Baird Publishing, London)
The Big Book of Juices and Smoothies Natalie Savona (Duncan Baird Publishing, London)
Books by Alice Waters, Hugh Fearnley-Whittingstall.

wonderfoods nutrient sources

NUTRIENTS PLAY A VITAL PART IN ALL THE WORKINGS OF THE HUMAN BODY, IN MAINTAINING GOOD HEALTH AND IN FIGHTING DISEASE. HERE IS A SUMMARY OF THE ROLES OF KEY NUTRIENTS AND WONDERFOODS YOU CAN EAT TO OBTAIN THEM.

Vitamin	Nutrient for...
Vitamin A/beta carotene	Antioxidant; protects skin and 'internal skin' – lungs, gut; eyes; reproduction; immunity
Vitamin B1	Energy production; nervous system; carbohydrate processing
Vitamin B2	Energy; skin; nervous system
Vitamin B3	Energy; nervous system; moods; blood sugar balance; cholesterol balance; stress response; hormonal balance
Vitamin B5	Energy production; body's stress response; regeneration of cells; anti-inflammatory; immunity
Vitamin B6	Energy production; nervous system; moods and brain power; hormone balance; protein digestion; immunity
Vitamin B12	Brain and nervous system; red blood cell formation; lowers toxic homocysteine; cellular energy and reproduction
Folic Acid	Brain and nervous system, especially in foetal growth; cellular energy and reproduction; moods; cardiovascular health; red blood cell formation; lowers toxic homocysteine
Biotin	Energy production; fat and amino acid processing; skin, nails and hair
Vitamin C	Antioxidant; collagen formation: skin, blood vessels and gums; aids iron absorption; immunity; helps protect against illness, allergies, pollution, stress and ageing; anti-inflammatory

Wonderfood Sources

Apricot, broccoli, carrot, kale, spinach, sweet potato, pumpkin, melon, watermelon, egg

Beans, sunflower seeds, fish, brown rice, oats, rye, quinoa, buckwheat, molasses, chicken, turkey, lamb, egg

Almonds, walnuts, Brazil nuts, oats, spinach, yoghurt, egg, fish, chicken, turkey, lamb

Chicken, turkey, lamb, fish, seeds, beans, lentils, soya, yoghurt

Egg, fish, chicken, turkey, lamb, brown rice, oats, rye, quinoa, buckwheat, lentils, soy

Chicken, turkey, lamb, fish, almonds, walnuts, Brazil nuts, brown rice, oats, rye, quinoa, buckwheat, avocado, banana, seeds, beans, lentils

Eggs, fish, chicken, turkey, lamb, yoghurt

All fruits, beans, lentils, soya, spinach, kale, parsley, oats, rye, quinoa, buckwheat

Egg, brown rice, oats, rye, quinoa, buckwheat, lentils, fish, seeds

Blackcurrants, berries, broccoli, cabbage, citrus fruit, sweet pepper, kale, kiwi fruit, papaya, spinach, tomato, watercress

Vitamin	Nutrient for...
Vitamin D	Helps calcium usage; bones and teeth; some cancer protection
Vitamin E	Antioxidant; immunity; helps protect skin, brain, circulation and hormones; cardiovascular system
Vitamin K	Blood clotting; bone building

Mineral	Nutrient for...
Calcium	Bone building; muscle contraction and relaxation; regular heart beat; blood clotting; nerve transmission
Chromium	Processing of carbohydrates and sugars; blood sugar balance; works with insulin
Copper	Production and transport of red blood cells; iron absorption; antioxidant
Iodine	Forms part of thyroid hormone
Iron	Forms part of haemoglobin i.e. helps transport oxygen; other uses include cell reproduction
Magnesium	Energy production; hormone balance; muscle and nerve function; cardiovascular health; blood sugar balance; works with calcium
Manganese	Antioxidant; energy production; nerves and brain; blood sugar balance; thyroid function
Potassium	Works with sodium to control fluid balance, blood pressure, nerves, muscles
Selenium	Antioxidant; works with vitamin E; immunity; cardiovascular health; anti-inflammatory

Wonderfood Sources

Fish, egg, yoghurt

Almonds, walnuts, Brazil nuts, seeds and seed oils, egg

Alfalfa sprouts, kale, parsley, spinach, broccoli, cauliflower, green tea

Wonderfood Sources

Almonds, Brazil nuts, walnuts, seeds, kale, spinach, broccoli, canned fish, yoghurt, molasses

Chicken, turkey, lamb, egg, fish, brown rice, oats, rye, quinoa, buckwheat, walnuts, almonds, Brazil nuts

Fish, walnuts, almonds, Brazil nuts, seeds, oats, rye, quinoa, buckwheat

Fish, seaweed

Egg, lamb, chicken, turkey, fish, prunes, seeds, seaweed, spinach, kale, brown rice, oats, rye, quinoa, buckwheat

Brown rice, oats, rye, quinoa, buckwheat, seeds, almonds, Brazil nuts, walnuts, molasses

Avocado, berries, buckwheat, ginger, hazelnuts, oats, seaweed, spinach

Avocado, banana, citrus fruit, lentils, nuts, sardines, spinach, whole grains

Fish, seeds, brown rice, oats, rye, quinoa, buckwheat, walnuts, Brazil nuts, almonds

Mineral	Nutrient for...
Sulphur	Antioxidant; helps liver detoxification; collagen production; skin, hair, nails
Zinc	Antioxidant; growth and development; all protein production; energy production; hormone production and balance; digestion; sexual function; skin health

Other essential nutrients	Nutrient for...
Essential Fatty Acids	As their name suggests, these are types of fats that the body cannot produce itself, so they must be obtained from food. They are needed for good hormone balance; healthy nerve and brain activities; smooth skin; cardiovascular health; they also have anti-inflammatory properties.
Protein	These are molecules made up of amino acids linked together in a particular order specified by a gene. They are needed for the structure, function and regulation of all the body's cells and organs. Hormones, neurotransmitters, enzymes, transporters and immune cells are proteins.
Carbohydrate	These are mainly sugars and starches that the body breaks down into glucose, a simple sugar used as fuel for the cells to make energy. They are found in sugar, all cereals, the wonderfoods listed opposite and other foods. The body also uses carbohydrate to make a substance called glycogen, which is stored in the body for future use.

Wonderfood Sources

Cabbage, egg, fish, garlic, onion

Egg, fish, chicken, turkey, lamb, seeds, yoghurt

Wonderfood Sources

Fish, seeds, nuts

Egg, fish, turkey, chicken, lamb, yoghurt, soya, nuts, seeds, beans, lentils

All fruit and vegetables, rice, buckwheat, oats, quinoa, rye, sweet potato, lentils, beans, honey

wonderfoods therapy

WE'RE ALL AWARE OF THE EFFECT THAT SOME FOODS AND DRINKS HAVE ON US: DRINK COFFEE AND YOU FEEL MORE ALERT, EAT TOO MUCH CAKE AND YOU FEEL BLOATED! AND THE SAME GOES FOR MANY COMMON AILMENTS — CERTAIN FOODS MAKE THEM WORSE WHILE SOME WONDERFOODS CAN HELP FIGHT, RELIEVE OR PREVENT THE SYMPTOMS. EATING THE FOODS SUGGESTED IS NOT INTENDED AS A REPLACEMENT FOR MEDICAL ADVICE.

Wonderfoods to eat

Acne

All fruit and vegetable fibre, oats, rye, brown rice, beans, lentils, beetroot, greens such as spinach, broccoli, watercress and kale, parsley, almonds, avocado, strawberries, mango, pumpkin, sweet potato, carrot, garlic, seeds, yoghurt

Anaemia

Greens such as spinach, broccoli, watercress and kale, parsley, beetroot, strawberries, kiwi fruit, citrus fruit, fish, egg, turkey, chicken, lamb, molasses

Arthritis

All fresh fruit and vegetables especially strawberries, blueberries, cherries, carrot, broccoli, watercress, kiwi fruit, apricot and pineapple, garlic, ginger, seeds and seed oils, fish, walnuts, Brazil nuts, prunes, turmeric, cinnamon

Asthma

All fresh fruit and vegetables especially blueberries, cherries, carrot, sweet pepper, broccoli, watercress and apricot, ginger, garlic, seeds and seed oils, fish, onion, pumpkin, sweet potato, walnuts

Bladder infection

Blueberries, watermelon, melon, broccoli, cherries, strawberries, kiwi fruit, citrus fruit, garlic, yoghurt

Boils

Blueberries, strawberries, watermelon, melon, kiwi fruit, citrus fruit, garlic, spinach, broccoli, watercress, kale, parsley, beetroot, artichoke, avocado, cucumber, almonds, mango, pumpkin, sweet potato, carrot

Bronchitis	Apricot, sweet pepper, watercress, watermelon, melon, blueberries, broccoli, strawberries, cherries, kiwi fruit, citrus fruit, garlic, seeds, pumpkin, sweet potato, onion, cloves
Burns, cuts & bruises	Apricot, sweet pepper, carrot, watercress, watermelon, melon, broccoli, strawberries, cherries, kiwi fruit, citrus fruit, garlic, seeds, mango, avocado, almonds, pumpkin, sweet potato
Candidiasis	Oats, rye, brown rice, beans, lentils, spinach, broccoli, watercress, kale, parsley, artichoke, beetroot, asparagus, dandelion, cucumber, yoghurt, garlic
Cardiovascular disease	All fruit and vegetable fibre, oats, rye, brown rice, beans, lentils, broccoli, strawberries, cherries, kiwi fruit, citrus fruit, celery, garlic, cucumber, grapes, seeds and seed oils, fish, turmeric, walnuts, Brazil nuts, prunes
Chronic fatigue	Greens such as spinach, broccoli, watercress and kale, parsley, strawberries, kiwi fruit, citrus fruit, yoghurt, egg, lamb, turkey, chicken, seeds and seed oils, fish, oats, buckwheat, seaweed
Cold sores	Watermelon, melon, broccoli, blueberries, strawberries, cherries, kiwi fruit, citrus fruit, garlic, carrot, sweet pepper, watercress, apricot, avocado, mango, pumpkin, sweet potato, garlic
Colitis	Watermelon, melon, broccoli, blueberries, strawberries, kiwi fruit, citrus fruit, garlic, carrot, sweet pepper, watercress, kale, apricot, pineapple, papaya, seeds and seed oils, fish, turmeric, cardamom
Common cold and flu	All fresh fruit and vegetables especially blueberries, carrot, apricot, broccoli, watercress, strawberries, kiwi fruit, pumpkin, sweet potato, onion and pineapple, ginger, garlic, seeds and seed oils, fish, Brazil nuts, cloves, cinnamon

Constipation	All fresh fruit and vegetables, prunes, oats, rye, brown rice, beans, lentils, seeds and seed oils, plenty of water and vegetable juices, dandelion, beetroot, artichoke, cucumber
Cystitis	Blueberries, watermelon, melon, broccoli, strawberries, kiwi fruit, citrus fruit, garlic, yoghurt
Depression	Yoghurt, egg, lamb, turkey, chicken, seeds and seed oils, fish, greens such as spinach, broccoli, watercress and kale, parsley, strawberries, kiwi fruit, citrus fruit, oats, quinoa, rye, walnuts, buckwheat
Dermatitis	All fresh fruit and vegetables especially berries, carrot, sweet pepper, apricot, broccoli, watercress, avocado, mango, pumpkin and sweet potato, almonds, ginger, garlic, seeds and seed oils, fish
Diabetes	All fruit and vegetable fibre, oats, rye, brown rice, beans, lentils, greens such as spinach, broccoli, watercress and kale, parsley, yoghurt, egg, turkey, chicken, seeds and seed oils, fish
Diarrhoea	Apple, carrot, celery (all cooked), white rice, plenty of water, yoghurt
Diverticulitis	All fruit and vegetable fibre, oats, rye, brown rice, beans, lentils, yoghurt, garlic, ginger, seed oils, fish, papaya, pineapple, cardamom
Dry skin	Berries, watermelon, melon, broccoli, kiwi fruit, garlic, carrot, sweet pepper, watercress, apricot, papaya, avocado, mango, walnuts, almonds, seeds and seed oils, fish
Ear infection	Blueberries, broccoli, strawberries, kiwi fruit, citrus fruit, garlic, onion, ginger, sweet potato, carrot, sweet pepper, apricot, watercress, kale, seeds and seed oils, fish

Eczema	Berries, cherries, carrot, sweet pepper, apricot, broccoli, watercress, avocado, mango, almonds, pumpkin, sweet potato, ginger, garlic, seeds and seed oils, fish, turmeric, walnuts, Brazil nuts, prunes
Fatigue	Sweet potato, pumpkin, banana, spinach, coconut, Jerusalem artichoke, honey, molasses, yoghurt, egg, turkey, chicken, seeds and seed oils, fish, lamb, seaweed, buckwheat
Fever	Fresh fruit and vegetable juices, blueberries, broccoli, strawberries, kiwi fruit, citrus fruit, garlic, carrot, sweet pepper, apricot, watercress, kale
Fibroids	All fruit and vegetable fibre, oats, rye, brown rice, beans, lentils, greens such as spinach, broccoli, watercress and kale, parsley, soya, seeds and seed oils, seaweed, celery
Gallbladder disorders	Apple, grapefruit, beetroot, dandelion, yoghurt, watercress, cardamom, kale, broccoli
Haemorrhoids	All fruit and vegetable fibre, oats, rye, brown rice, beans, lentils, blueberries, broccoli, strawberries, kiwi fruit, citrus fruit, buckwheat
Hangovers	Carrot, celery, apple, ginger, spinach, broccoli, watercress, kale, parsley, yoghurt, garlic, onion, cardamom, pineapple, artichoke, cucumber
Hay fever	All fresh fruit and vegetables especially blueberries, cherries, carrot, sweet pepper, apricot, broccoli and watercress, ginger, garlic, seeds and seed oils, fish
Heartburn	Pineapple, papaya, cabbage, dandelion, cardamom, ginger
Herpes	Watermelon, melon, blueberries, strawberries, cherries, carrot, sweet potato, broccoli, kiwi fruit, citrus fruit, avocado, garlic, yoghurt

High blood pressure	*All fruit and vegetable fibre, oats, rye, brown rice, beans, lentils, broccoli, strawberries, kiwi fruit, citrus fruit, seeds and seed oils, fish, celery, cucumber, garlic, grapes, cinnamon*
Hypothyroid	*Seaweed, seeds and seed oils, fish*
Indigestion	*Pineapple, papaya, cabbage, ginger, cardamom*
Irritable bowel syndrome	*Pineapple, papaya, cabbage, dandelion, fresh vegetable juices, spinach, broccoli, watercress, kale, parsley, yoghurt, garlic, onion, ginger, cardamom, pineapple, artichoke, celery, cucumber, yoghurt*
Memory problems	*Seeds and seed oils, fish, thyme, egg, strawberries, blueberries, watermelon, melon, broccoli, kiwi fruit, citrus fruit, turmeric, walnuts*
Menopause-related problems	*All fruit and vegetable fibre, oats, rye, brown rice, beans, lentils, greens such as spinach, broccoli, watercress and kale, parsley, soya, seeds and seed oils, seaweed, celery*
Muscle cramps	*Spinach, broccoli, watercress, kale, parsley, yoghurt, garlic, molasses, seeds, buckwheat*
Osteoporosis	*Spinach, broccoli, watercress, kale, parsley, yoghurt, garlic, molasses, seeds, buckwheat*
Premenstrual syndrome	*All fruit and vegetable fibre, oats, rye, brown rice, beans, lentils, greens such as spinach, broccoli, watercress and kale, parsley, soya, seeds and seed oils, seaweed, celery*
Prostate problems	*Tomato, pumpkin seeds, all fruit and vegetable fibre, oats, rye, brown rice, beans, lentils, greens such as spinach, broccoli, watercress and kale, parsley, soya, seeds and seed oils, celery*

Psoriasis	Berries, cherries, carrot, sweet pepper, broccoli, watercress, avocado, apricot, almonds, mango, pumpkin, sweet potato, ginger, garlic, seeds and seed oils, fish, turmeric, walnuts, Brazil nuts, prunes
Sinusitis	All fresh fruit and vegetables especially blueberries, strawberries, carrot, apricot, broccoli, watercress, kiwi fruit, pineapple and onion, ginger, garlic, seeds and seed oils, fish
Sleeping problems	Spinach, broccoli, watercress, kale, parsley, yoghurt, seeds, buckwheat, banana
Sprains, strains & other injuries	Spinach, broccoli, watercress, kale, parsley, cherries, pineapple, papaya, seeds and seed oils, garlic, molasses, turmeric, ginger
Stress	Yoghurt, egg, lamb, turkey, chicken, seeds and seed oils, fish, spinach, broccoli, watercress, kale, parsley, strawberries, kiwi fruit, citrus fruit, oats, quinoa, rye
Tonsillitis	Broccoli, blueberries, strawberries, cherries, kiwi fruit, citrus fruit, garlic, onion, ginger, sweet potato, carrot, sweet pepper, apricot, watercress, kale, seeds and seed oils, fish
Varicose veins	All fruit and vegetable fibre, oats, rye, brown rice, beans, lentils, blueberries, strawberries, cherries, kiwi fruit, citrus fruit, broccoli, seeds and seed oils, fish, garlic, ginger, buckwheat, turmeric, prunes, herbs

wonderfoods glossary

amino acid The building blocks of proteins in our food and throughout the body.

anthocyanidins Powerful antioxidant chemicals found in some plants, particularly blue, red and purple ones.

antihistamine A substance that counteracts the action of the inflammatory, allergic body chemical histamine.

antioxidant A substance or enzyme that neutralises oxidants, or free radicals, protecting cells from damage that can lead to disease and ageing.

bacteria Minute, single-celled organisms that live in us and in the environment. Some are harmful and others are beneficial.

bile Fluid produced by the liver to help digestion, particularly of fats, and the elimination of waste products.

bioflavonoids Antioxidant chemicals found in some foods.

cardiovascular disease An umbrella term for a range of conditions affecting the heart and blood vessels such as high blood pressure, atherosclerosis (hardening of the arteries) and high cholesterol.

carotenoids A family of colourful compounds found in foods with antioxidant properties that are considered to be plant forms of vitamin A.

chlorophyll The green pigment in plants, which they need to capture sunlight in order to produce energy.

cholesterol A fat-like substance found in some foods, produced in the liver and present throughout the human body. It's needed in the body, in cell structure for example, and for making some hormones. In excess, it can be a harmful component of cardiovascular disease, particularly when oxidised.

complex carbohydrate Starches and fibre in foods that have not been refined; the starches can be broken down to produce energy.

detoxification The body's natural 'cleansing' processes by which it clears waste products and eliminates them.

diuretic A substance which increases the rate of urination, promoting loss of water from the body.

enzyme A protein which acts as a catalyst in any of the countless processes in the body. The term is also used to describe substances that help the breakdown of foods in the gut.

essential fatty acids (EFAs) Fats, such as those found in fish, nuts and seeds, that are a necessary part of our diet for good health.

fibre A part of foods, especially fruit, vegetables and whole grains, that the human gut cannot digest. Fibre helps slow down the release of digested food as glucose into the bloodstream, bulks out the stool, feeds beneficial bacteria and encourages the elimination of waste products.

flavonoids A family of antioxidant chemicals found in some plants.

free radical An oxidant, an atom that is unstable and stabilises itself by robbing a nearby molecule, thereby creating a cascade of oxidative damage. This process is a normal part of cell workings, but in excess, is linked to ageing, heart disease, cancer and other chronic diseases.

fructo-oligo-saccharides (FOS) Indigestible, sweet-tasting, soluble fibre found in some foods that can be used as fuel by the beneficial bacteria in our intestines.

GLA (gamma linoleic acid) A fatty acid needed for healthy hormone balance, to help lower inflammation and to reduce blood clotting. GLA is found in some plants (borage, for example) and in evening primrose oil. It can also be made in the body as a derivative from linoleic acid (found in seeds such as sunflower).

glucosinolates Chemicals naturally found in some foods, especially the brassica family (broccoli, cabbage, kale etc.) that help the liver's detoxification processes and act as antioxidants.

harissa This is a North African spice paste. If unobtainable, use a sprinkling of paprika and a dash of Tabasco sauce instead.

hormone Produced in a gland, this is a chemical messenger that travels via blood to sites elsewhere in the body to transmit its specific 'message' to cells. Examples are thyroxine (regulates growth and metabolism) and oestrogen (the female sex and reproduction hormone).

immune system The body's complex collection of means for protecting against harmful organisms and fighting them once they are in the body.

insulin The hormone produced by the pancreas whose most important role is to help sugar (glucose) get into cells to make energy.

isoflavones Chemicals found in some plants, such as soya, that can have oestrogen-like effects in the body.

medium chain triglycerides (MCTs) Fats found in some foods, such as coconut, that are easily absorbed and used to make energy, and appear to help boost metabolism.

mineral Natural inorganic substance, such as iron and magnesium, also called metal. Minerals are found in the earth, in food and in our bodies, where they form part of the structure and function.

miso A Japanese, fermented soya paste used to make soups.

monounsaturated fats A type of fat, such as that found in olive oil, which has a chemical structure that makes it useful in the body and is linked to good health.

mucous membrane The lubricated lining of passages in the body that open up to the 'outside world' i.e. the digestive tract, vagina and respiratory system.

neurotransmitter A chemical messenger molecule used in the nervous system to convey messages, such as those for memory or mood, between one cell and another.

omega 3 fats A family of fats (found in oily fish, flax seeds and walnuts, for example) essential for healthy skin, brain, nerves, hormones and cardiovascular health, as well as lowering inflammation.

omega 6 fats A family of fats (found in sunflower and pumpkin seeds, for example) that are needed in the body for healthy skin, hormones and for lowering inflammation.

oxidant A naturally occurring, unstable molecule which, if left unchecked by sufficient antioxidants, can cause damage to cells. Also known as a free radical.

pectin A type of soluble fibre that is found in some fruits, such as apples, pears and citrus fruit.

prebiotic Fibre, such as that found in Jerusalem artichokes, which is useful for feeding the beneficial bacteria in the gut.

probiotic A term used to describe beneficial bacteria that we can get from quality yoghurt or in a capsule, which replenishes those we have living in our intestines.

protein Large molecules made up of specific chains of amino acids that are used in and make up the body. They are vital for structure, enzymes, neurotransmitters and transport in the body.

saturated fat (SF) Fats found in animal-derived foods such as milk, cheese, yoghurt and meat which, in excess, is linked to cardiovascular disease. Coconut and palm oils also contain saturated fat.

serotonin A neurotransmitter made and used in the body, associated with good moods and sleep amongst other things.

tahini A paste made purely from crushed sesame seeds.

tamari A wheat-free sauce made from the fermentation of soya beans, similar to soy sauce.

tryptophan An amino acid that the body can use to make vitamin B3 and serotonin and needed for growth.

vitamin An organic micronutrient found in foods that is vital to health, normal body processes and disease prevention.

Index

Acknowledgements

My thanks to...Barbara Levy for always being there, on my team, Anne Furniss with whom
I shared the idea of Wonderfoods over a great salad and a coffee, Jill Mead whose evocative
photography leaves words in the shade, Janet Illsley for expertly knocking my words into
shape and Ros Holder for making the whole thing look gorgeous. And to my friends who
risked testing recipes: Theresa Banovic, Robert Brennan, Janet Kipling, Marion and Bob Luker.
Also, to my Maltese family cooking greats – Nanna, Auntie Marlene and Auntie Claire, Arielle
who's not only a fellow piggy but is the best sister ever, and my parents who have always
lavished me with love and good food. And to A, who nourishes my tummy and the rest, not
forgetting my dog Splash, my bees, my computer doctor and anyone else I've overlooked...